T0320570

# NEW TECHNOLOGIES FOR RECLAMATION OF INDUSTRIAL WASTEWATER

# NEW TECHNOLOGIES FOR RECLAMATION OF INDUSTRIAL WASTEWATER

### Authored By

Pankaj Chowdhary and Sujata Mani

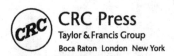

**CRC Press**
Taylor & Francis Group
Boca Raton  London  New York

CRC Press is an imprint of the
Taylor & Francis Group, an **informa** business

First edition published 2021
by CRC Press
6000 Broken Sound Parkway NW, Suite 300, Boca Raton, FL 33487-2742

and by CRC Press
2 Park Square, Milton Park, Abingdon, Oxon, OX14 4RN

© 2021 Taylor & Francis Group, LLC

CRC Press is an imprint of Taylor & Francis Group, LLC

*Library of Congress Cataloging-in-Publication Data*
Names: Chowdhary, Pankaj, author. | Mani, Sujata, author.
Title: New technologies for reclamation of industrial wastewater / authored
by Pankaj Chowdhary and Sujata Mani.
Description: First edition. | Boca Raton : CRC Press, 2021. | Includes
bibliographical references and index.
Identifiers: LCCN 2020044929 | ISBN 9780367434182 (hardback) | ISBN
9781003003281 (ebook)
Subjects: LCSH: Sewage--Purification. | Factory and trade
waste--Purification. | Water--Pollution. | Environmental toxicology.
Classification: LCC TD745 .C38 2021 | DDC 628.4/3--dc23
LC record available at https://lccn.loc.gov/2020044929

ISBN: 978-0-367-43418-2 (hbk)
ISBN: 978-0-367-70414-8 (pbk)
ISBN: 978-1-003-00328-1 (ebk)

Typeset in Times New Roman
by MPS Limited, Dehradun

# Contents

# Abbreviations

| | |
|---|---|
| **AGP** | Algal Growth Potential |
| **AOP** | Advance Oxidation Process |
| **AOX** | Absorbable Organic Halides |
| **AS** | Activated Sludge |
| **BAA** | Bromoamine Acid |
| **BCTMP** | Bleaching of Thermo-Mechanical Pulp |
| **BOD** | Biological Oxygen Demand |
| **C/N** | Carbon/Nitrogen |
| **COD** | Chemical Oxygen Demand |
| **CPCB** | Central Pollution Control Board |
| **Da** | Dalton |
| **DBP** | Dibutyl Phthalate |
| **DGBE** | Diethylene Glycol Monobutyl Ether |
| **DO** | Dissolved Oxygen |
| **EDC** | Endocrine Disrupting Compound |
| **EGSB** | Expanded Granular Sludge Bed |
| **ETP** | Effluent Treatment Plant |
| **FBBR** | Fluidized Bed Biofilm Reactor |
| **GC/MS** | Gas Chromatography/Mass Spectrometry |
| **MBR** | Membrane Batch Reactor |
| **MCL** | Maximum Contaminant Level |
| **MF** | Microfiltration |
| **MSW** | Molasses Spent Wash |
| **NP** | Nonylphenol |
| **NPE** | Nonylethoxyphenol |
| **P&P** | Pulp and Paper |
| **PAH** | Polycyclic Aromatic Hydrocarbon |
| **PCB** | Poly Chlorinated Biphenyls |
| **PhAC** | Pharmaceutically Active Compound |
| **POP** | Persistent Organic Pollutants |
| **PPM** | Parts Per Million |
| **PVA** | Polyvinyl Alcohol |
| **QS** | Quorum Sensing |
| **R&D** | Research and Development |

| | |
|---|---|
| **RBC** | Rotating Biological Contactor |
| **RO** | Reverse Osmosis |
| **ROP** | Recalcitrant Organic Pollutants |
| **SBR** | Sequence Batch Reactor |
| **SOC** | Synthetic Organic Compounds |
| **TDS** | Total Dissolved Solid |
| **TMP** | Thermo-mechanical Pulping |
| **TOC** | Total Organic Carbon |
| **TSS** | Total Suspended Solid |
| **UF** | Ultra-filtration |
| **WHO** | World Health Organization |
| **WWTP** | Wastewater Treatment Plant |

# Author Biographies

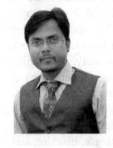 **Dr. Pankaj Chowdhary** is President, Society for Green Environment (SGE) at New Delhi, India. He completed his Ph.D. (2018) in Microbiology from the Department of Environmental Microbiology at Babasaheb Bhimrao Ambedkar University, Lucknow, Uttar Pradesh, India. His doctorate work was focused on the role of ligninolytic enzyme producing bacterial strains in the decolorizing & degradation of coloring compounds from distillery wastewater. His main research areas are Microbial Biotechnology, Biodegradation and Bioremediation of Environmental contaminants in Industrial wastewaters, Metagenomics and Lignocellulosic waste valorization. He has edited three books, including *Emerging and Eco-friendly Approaches for Waste Management, Contaminants and Clean Technologies* and *Microorganisms for Sustainable Environment and Health*. In addition, he has authored two books, *New Technologies for Reclamation of Industrial Wastewater* and *Recent Advances in Distillery Waste Management for Environmental Safety*. Dr. Chowdhary has published many research/review papers in national and international peer-reviewed journals of high impact factor published by Springer, Elsevier, Royal Society of Chemistry (RSC), Taylor & Francis Group and Frontiers. He has also published many national and international book chapters and magazine articles on the biodegradation and bioremediation of environmental pollutants, presented many posters/papers relevant to research areas at conferences around the world, and actively worked as a potential reviewer in various SCI-journals published from reputed international publishers (Springer, Elsevier, Royal Society of Chemistry (RSC), Taylor & Francis Group, Wiley and Frontiers). He is a lifetime member of the Association of Microbiologists of India (AMI) and Indian Science Congress Association (ISCA), Kolkata, India.

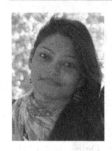 **Dr. Sujata Mani** is currently working as an Assistant Professor and actively engaged in teaching and research activities at the Department of Biochemistry, Gramin Science Vocational College, Vishnupuri, Nanded, Maharashtra, India. She completed her Ph.D. degree in Microbiology from Babasaheb Bhimrao Ambedkar Central University, Lucknow, Uttar Pradesh, India in 2018. During her Ph.D. she was awarded with Rajiv Gandhi National Fellowship (Both JRF and SRF). Her doctorate work was focused on degradation and detoxification mechanism of crystal violet from textile wastewater for environmental safety. Her major areas of research were biodegradation and bioremediation of synthetic dyes in textile wastewater through bacterial species producing ligninolytic enzymes. She has published review/research papers in reputed national and international journals with high impact factors. She has also published many book chapters in national and international edited books published by Springer, Elsevier, and Taylor & Francis Group. She is also a qualified ICAR-NET in Microbiology. She has also guided graduate and postgraduate dissertation students. She is a life member of the Association of Microbiologists of India (AMI) and Indian Science Congress Association (ISCA), Kolkata, India.

# Acknowledgments

The authors would like to express their sincere thanks to the all supports and well-wishers, especially Mr. Anil Kumar Singh, AcSIR Ph.D. (UGC-SRF), for figures preparation and other scientific assistance. Dr. Chowdhary acknowledges the support received from his family, especially his father (Mr. Ram Chandra) and mother (Mrs. Malti Devi). Dr. Mani acknowledges the support of her father (Mr. Chandra Mani), mother (Mrs. Gayatri Devi), and husband (Mr. Ankush Teshwar). The authors also acknowledge the cooperation received from the CRC publishing team at Taylor & Francis and for their guidance in finalizing this book.

# General Introduction of Industries

# 1

Industrialization, although it plays a vital role in the development and establishment of a country's economy, has now become the major source of environmental pollution throughout the world. Nowadays, the major concern of the researchers and scientists dealing the preservation problems is the waste discharge from various industries, since they consist of a variety of pollutants (organic and inorganic) and highly toxic heavy metals. These toxic pollutants cause severe water and soil pollution. If, by chance, it reaches humans and animals through accumulation, it can cause numerous fatal diseases such as delayed nervous disorders, neurological disorders, mutagenic changes, cancer, etc. Treatment of discharged wastewater is essential for environmental as well as human safety. There are various treatment processes such as physical, chemical, and biological methods that have been reported with regards to discharge of industrial effluents into the environment. The main problem with the physico-chemical treatment processes, aside from its excessive cost, are the large amount of sludge generated which acts as secondary pollutant. Biological processes—being of simple structural set-up—are cost-effective, easy to operate, has extensive application and diverse metabolic pathways, environmental-friendly with the versatility of microorganisms, and has less production of sludge in comparison to physico-chemical methods. Based on these advantages, biological methods using microbes are becoming extremely popular among various existing industrial wastewater treatment processes.

## 1.1 TYPES OF INDUSTRIAL EFFLUENTS AND THEIR CHARACTERISTICS

The types of industrial wastewaters are described based on their source of industrial origin,—tannery, textile, distillery, pulp and paper, electroplating,

1

iron and steel mine, pharmaceuticals, etc. Each industry discharges a different type of pollutant or contaminant with the wastewaters into the environment. The textile industry releases various coloring dyes and other toxic organic and inorganic pollutants along with wastewater (Ahmad et al., 2020). Similarly, petrochemical industries release mineral oils and phenols; pulp and paper industries release chlorine-based substances, suspended solids, and organic materials. Like this, various industries release other types of pollutants; therefore, specific treatment must be designed for a particular type of pollutant produced in the wastewater (Singh et al., 2016). Different industrial sectors and their released pollutants have been described in Table 1.1. Usually, industrial effluents are categorized into two types: organic and inorganic.

## 1.1.1 Organic Industrial Effluent

Large-scale chemical industries that use organic substances for chemical reactions have been categorized under organic industrial effluents. These organic pollutants can be removed through pre-treatment of the wastewater with a combination of biological treatment methods. Most of the organic pollutants in the wastewater are produced from tannery or leather industries, textile industries, paper and cellulose producing factories, oil refineries, pharmaceutical industries, metal processing factories, etc. The production of wastes from these industries comes from the different use of raw materials, their working methods, and generated waste products. Due to various product manufacturing in the same industry, it gives rise to pollutants from different production processes. The wastewater generated has low $BOD_5$ concentration with high COD concentration, and their ratio is lower than 30%, showing poor biodegradability of wastewater. Some effluents show high pH with lousy odor and color. Thus, various treatment processes are required at different stages of industrial product manufacture.

## 1.1.2 Inorganic Industrial Effluent

These types of wastewaters are produced from industries like coal and steel, non-metallic mineral, iron, and electroplating, etc. The effluents generated consist of massive quantities of suspended materials that are eradicated through a combination of sedimentation and chemical flocculation treatment process with the addition of aluminum or iron salts. The wastewaters with dissolved and undissolved inorganic substances come from the release of dust-laden wastes from aluminum works, blast furnaces, converters, cupola furnaces, trash, and slurry incineration plants. Approximately 2 $m^3$ tons of

**TABLE 1.1** Industrial sectors and their water pollutants

| S. no. | Industrial sectors | Water pollutants |
|---|---|---|
| 1. | Chemical Industry | High COD, heavy metals, organic chemicals, cyanide, suspended solids, etc. |
| 2. | Distillery Industry | High BOD & COD, high suspended solids, melanoidins, chemicals, organic and inorganic materials, etc. |
| 3. | Food Industry | High suspended solids, organic materials, sulfides, mineral oil, mercaptans, emulsified fat, chemicals, amines, etc. |
| 4. | Iron and Steel Industry | High BOD & COD, metals, oil, acids, cyanide, phenols, etc. |
| 5. | Mining | Acids, metals, suspended solids, salts, etc. |
| 6. | Micro-electronics | Organic chemicals, high COD, electronic waste products, etc. |
| 7. | Non-ferrous metals | Fluorine, suspended solids, etc. |
| 8. | Petrochemicals | High BOD and COD range, chromium, mineral oil, phenols, etc. |
| 9. | Pharmaceuticals | Chemicals, natural and synthetic solvents, organic wastes, High COD, low BOD, etc. |
| 10. | Pulp and Paper | Chloride organics, dioxins, suspended solids, organic materials or wastes, $SO_2$ etc. |
| 11. | Tannery Industry | High BOD, suspended and dissolved solids, chromium, sulfates, high chloride, emulsified fat, etc. |
| 12. | Textile Industry | High BOD & COD, variety of synthetic dyes, metals, organic and inorganic chemicals, suspended as well as dissolved solids, etc. |

water is required during pre-cooling and subsequent purification of blast furnace gases. During this process, water in the gas cooler absorbs fine particles of coke, iron, and more along with some metals which don't get settle down and are washed out with the water. Other types of wastewaters, like the ones from rolling mills, contain mineral oils that require additional setup of scum boards to skim-off their preservation and removal from discharged effluents. The non-metallic mineral and metal processing plants should treat and purify their effluents before its release into municipal wastewater systems in acquiescence with local regulations.

# 1.2 CHARACTERISTICS OF INDUSTRIAL EFFLUENTS

The characteristics of wastewater discharge depend on the different production processes, raw materials, and value of the product of the industries that discharge them. The industrial effluents are mainly characterized based on the high level of BOD, COD, TDS, TSS, various toxic metals, presence of a variety of organic and inorganic pollutants such as lignin, melanoidins, dyes, PHAs, etc. These characteristics (physical, chemical, and biological) of wastewaters will be described in this section.

## 1.2.1 Physical Characteristics

The flavor or aesthetic adequacy of the water for personal, agricultural, and domestic purposes are included under physical characteristics of effluents, and usually respond to the sense of smell, sight, taste, or touch. Some of these characteristics are color, odor, temperature, and solid contents, which will be described below.

### 1.2.1.1 Color

The universal condition for determining any industrial wastewaters is its color immediately after being discharged from any industry. If the color of the wastewater is light brown, it means that it has been discharged before six hours. Wastewater from light to medium grey shows that wastewater has undergone some process of decomposition or has been in the collection tank for a long time; dark grey or black color shows that it has extensively undergone a bacterial decomposition process under aerobic conditions. The black color of the wastewater is associated with sulfide formations—mostly ferrous sulfide—that result due to the production of hydrogen sulfide under anaerobic conditions in combination with divalent metals.

### 1.2.1.2 Odor

The odor from the wastewater determines its degree of treatment and is particularly important. When compared, the odor of the freshwater is not as strong as the industrial wastewaters. The different pungent odors such as ammonia, amines, fermentation, $H_2S$, sulfides, etc., are produced due to decomposition, as these wastewaters are generated from different industries such as food, textile, distillery, rubber, pulp and paper, tannery, pharmaceuticals, etc. (Brault and Degrement, 1991). The successive dilutions of the samples quantify odor and is done until there is no significant difference when compared with odor-free fresh water.

### 1.2.1.3 Temperature

The temperature of industrial wastewater is comparatively higher than that of regular water. It is also established that the temperature of the industrial wastewater varies with the topographical locations of the industries. According to Crites and Tchobanoglous (1998), in colder regions, the temperature of the wastewaters varies from 7 to 18 °C, while in warmer regions, it varies from 13 to 30 °C. Before subjecting to any treatment, the temperature of the wastewater should be measured since most treatment methods are temperature dependent.

### 1.2.1.4 Solid Contents

The total aggregate of soluble and insoluble materials in industrial wastewaters is considered as solid content. In most industrial wastewaters, the average discharge of 40–65% are the suspended solids (Crites and Tchobanoglous, 1998). The solids have been categorized into volatile solids—which easily get vaporized at hot temperatures of 600 °C—and fixed solids that do not get vaporized at any temperature. Volatile solids are usually assumed to be both organic matter—comprised mainly of carbohydrates, fats, and proteins that break at high temperatures but do not easily burn—and inorganic salts that break down at high temperatures.

## 1.2.2 Chemical Characteristics

The chemical characteristics of the industrial wastewaters depend on the raw materials, chemicals, procedures, and products. The wastewater's chemical natures are analyzed through principal chemical tests, which are based on free ammonia, organic and inorganic phosphorus, organic nitrogen, nitrates, and nitrites. The discharged wastewater consists of an elevated level of toxic metals, recalcitrant compounds, nutrients, organic and inorganic materials, etc. The heavy metals discharged along with the wastewater can produce toxic effects on the ecosystem; therefore, it is crucial to determine and evaluate their amount in the treated effluent. Other heavy metals such as chromium, arsenic, mercury, cadmium, etc., are considered as priority pollutants and must be removed from the effluent before its discharge into the environment

(Hare et al., 2019, 2020). Two nutrients—nitrogen and phosphorus—are responsible for the growth of aquatic plants, so their level should be monitored in the treated wastewater before their discharge into any body of water (Rein, 2005). The most common soil pollutants in industrialized wastewater are volatile organic compounds, which include toluene, xylenes, benzene, dichloromethane, trichloroethane, and trichloroethylene. However, there are other organic compounds that are now included in the list of priority pollutants like PCBs, acetaldehyde, formaldehyde, 1,2-dichloroethane, hexachlorobenzene, etc. (Bond and Straub, 1974).

### 1.2.3 Biological Characteristics

The biological characteristics include the estimation of pathogenic and non-pathogenic microorganisms, the oxygen demand by these microbes, and the level of organic pollutants in the industrial wastewater. The measurement of oxygen demand—aerobic and anaerobic bacteria, fungi, actinomycetes, viruses, and yeasts—is done in terms of biological oxygen demand or chemical oxygen demand.

# 1.3 WASTEWATER-PRODUCING INDUSTRIES

Industrial sources are the primary cause for the generation of toxic contaminants into aquatic wastewater systems. There are millions of industries, mills, and factories that discharge of toxic and hazardous pollutants all around the world (Dsikowitzky and Schwarzbauer, 2013) without treatment. Industrial wastes are categorized into biodegradable and non-biodegradable wastes—which are composed of organic and inorganic chemicals, corrosives, toxic liquids and solids, pesticides, hazardous metals, etc. which are generated from some of the industries described below.

## 1.3.1 Wastewater Produced from Tannery Industry

The tannery industry, which has been now labeled as "red category industry," is the biggest producer of leather—and has one of the most contaminated wastewaters. This industry has been the oldest when it comes to producing valuable leather items by using raw skin and hides, but their process utilizes large volumes of fresh water (i.e., ~35-40 L), most of which are discharged as wastewater containing pollutants (Chowdhary et al., 2013). The processing of raw skins and hides involves several steps and releases water with different hides, chemical, and mechanical methods used during the tanning process. The percentage of the wastewaters released during tanning processes are given as below:

- Bark tanning: 2.0%
- Chrome tanning: 2.0%
- Liming: 17.5%
- Plumping and bating: 19.0%
- Rinsing: 5.5%
- Soaking and washing: 22.5%
- Washing and drumming: 31.5%

After processing, the wastewaters released have high concentrations of COD (1,500–2,500 mg/L), high chlorine content (5 g/L) with acidic pH, emulsified fat, high settleable substances (10–20 g/L) with foam forming tendency. Along with this, wastewater also consists of chlorides, sulfates, colored complexes, toxic metals (chromium), and many other pollutants that are toxic to the ecosystem and health.

# 1.3.2 Wastewater Produced from the Textile Industry

Textile industries are the largest consumer of fresh water at ~30–50 L/kg during processing methods. Using several types of dyes, pigments, and various organic and inorganic chemicals that are discharged as pollutants after processing, it creates a vast environmental pollution problem. During the manufacturing of textile products, it is estimated that ~700,000 tons of numerous kinds of dyes—as well as 8,000 or more types of chemicals—are used in clothing, dying, and textile industries (Mani and Bharagava, 2016). The wastewaters generated during the processing from these industries are very dark in color, comprised of chlorine residues, dioxins, toxic heavy metals, and reactive dyes, pesticides, persistent organic pollutants (POP's), etc. (Zollinger, 1987). The dark color of the textile industrial wastewater is due to the extensive utilization of pigmented raw materials and dyes, and effluents have high BOD and total dissolved solids. When these toxic effluents are directly discharged into the environment without proper treatment, it can cause worsening of freshwater bodies as well as soil properties, which could be very harmful to animals, plants, and mankind.

The World Health Organization (WHO) approximated that 1–20% of total industrial wastewaters containing toxic and hazardous organic and inorganic wastes from textile industries cause significant environmental contamination and pollution (HSRC, 2005). In textile industries, 60–70% of the synthetic dyes utilized are being used as a regular dyestuff, which is highly toxic and exceedingly difficult to decolorize as well as degrade because of their complex structures. Some of these synthetic dyes and their intermediate compounds—which are mutagenic and carcinogenic in nature—are aromatic compounds, benzidine, naphthalene, etc. These compounds cause deleterious effects on humans, crops, and photosynthetic entities (Anjaneyulu et al., 2005).

## 1.3.3 Wastewater Produced from the Pharmaceutical Industry

The quality of wastewater generated from pharmaceutical industries and companies depends on the raw materials utilized for production and postproduction. The characteristics of the effluents vary from other industrial wastewaters as most of the products are manufactured in the same pharmaceutical plant at the same time. Therefore, the effluent generated is from diverse manufacturing zones. At a large scale, it is usual that along with the desired pharmaceutical manufactured products, several other chemical products can be yielded that include extracted residues of synthetic or natural solvents, various poisonous and hazardous substances, organic and inorganic compounds, dyes, recalcitrant heavy metals, etc. The wastewaters generated from pharmaceutical industries, if not appropriately treated, can lead to exceedingly high COD concentration (i.e., ~5000–15,000 mg/L) and low $BOD_5$ concentrations. The ration of $BOD_5$ to COD is lower than 30%, depicting the low biodegradability of the wastewater. This type of wastewater has a powerful odor with an extreme pH level and needs a strong treatment followed by biological treatments for an exceedingly long time.

## 1.3.4 Wastewater Produced from Distillery Industry

Alcohols are widely used in the production of cosmetics, chemicals, food, pharmaceuticals, perfume industries, etc., and has led to an increased establishment of alcohol-producing industries. Distillery industries produce ~8–15 L of wastewater per total liquor produced. In India, ~300 molasses-based industries have been reported, which produces ~40 billion liters of effluents annually. Since molasses are cheap, they are used as raw materials in most alcohol-producing industries, and the waste generated from these is known as a molasses-spent wash (MSW). MSW consists of melanoidins—a complex polymeric compound distributing a deep brown color to the wastewaters generated (Chowdhary et al., 2018a, b, 2020b, c). MSW has high concentrations of chemical oxygen demand COD (80,000–160,000 mg/L), mineral salts, phenols, organic compounds, low pH (3.7–4.5), dissolved solids, and low rate of biodegradability—which is a serious environmental problem. Melanoidins released along with the wastewaters are very toxic in nature, which leads to high levels of soil pollution in agricultural lands by causing manganese deficiency, reduction in soil alkalinity, inhibition in seed germination, and ultimately damaging the crops (Boudh et al., 2020). When these wastewaters are released in freshwater bodies, they cause eutrophication, acidification, and even interrupts the photosynthetic activities of the aquatic flora and fauna (Chowdhary et al., 2017c). The large generation of toxic and recalcitrant compounds containing wastewaters into the environment shows lethal effects on soil microbial communities as well as on aquatic microorganisms and animals (Pant and Adholeya, 2007b).

## 1.3.5 Wastewater Produced from the Brewery Industry

One of the grains used in the brewery industry is barley, which is used to brew beer with oats, rice, wheat, rye, and millet. Production of beer involves three steps: malt preparation from barley, wort preparation, and finally, fermentation by adding yeast. These processes are involved in the production of wastewaters, which are generated while washing and cleaning the barley, machines, filters, and containers like barrels and bottles. The wastewaters generated are high in detergents and suspended solids, while other parts of the wastewaters are due to the fermentation process—which has high concentrations of both $BOD_5$ and COD due to soluble and insoluble organic compounds. It is reported that the concentration of brewery wastewater is three to four times higher than sewage wastewaters; however, no toxic substances are found in the brewery wastewaters. Other organic compounds reported in wastewater are found to be biodegradable. Therefore, after removing the suspended solids through anaerobic biological treatment processes, the concentration of organic substances is automatically reduced. Finally, the quality of the wastewaters discharged can match the standards by following the aerobic biological treatment methods.

## 1.3.6 Wastewater Produced from Pulp and Paper Industry

Pulp and paper industrial effluents are rich in Recalcitrant Organic Pollutants (ROPs) because of the utilization of different chemicals during processing, causing a serious threat to our environment. The high amount of water (~4000–12,000 gal per tons of pulp) as well as high energy is required during the processing steps—out of which, ~75% of water is re-fluxed as wastewater (Ince et al., 2011). The production of paper takes place with two main steps: one is pulping and the other is bleaching; the pulping phase is the major source of toxic pollutants. The effluents generated from these industries consist of remarkably high concentrations of toxic and recalcitrant pollutants, which are continuously being released into the environment every year without proper treatment. The effluent consists of high concentration of salts and acids (calcium, carbonates, sodium, sulfide, $Na(OH)$, $Na_2CO_3$, $Ca(OH)_2$, $Na_2S$, $HCl$, $HNO_3$, $H_2SO_4$), chlorinated organic and inorganic compounds, nutrients, heavy metals, and various gases including NOx—which are emitted into the air, contaminating the soil, air, and water ecosystems. These pollutants are accumulated into our food chain, which is difficult to degrade due to their reactivity and structure complexity. These can cause severe neural impairments, cancer, and physiological health problems that is of significant concern for our society (Ince et al., 2011).

# 1.4 MAJOR POLLUTANTS IN INDUSTRIAL WASTEWATERS

The characteristics of the wastewaters released depend on the nature, amount of water, and chemicals utilized during the different manufacturing processes of different industries. The wastewaters released from different industries are highly composite in nature, consisting of a variety of organic and inorganic recalcitrant compounds, toxic heavy metals, dissolved, and suspended solids. Most of the industries use an assortment of chemicals at different processing stages such as bleaching agents, chlorides, chlorinated compounds, dye kinds of stuff, finishing chemicals, phenolic compounds, hypochlorite, organic and inorganic compounds, various metal salts such as Cr, Cu, Hg, Ni, Zn, etc. (Dey and Islam, 2015). Among the harmful compounds used in industries, phenolic compounds give unpleasant odor due to the frequency and toxicity generated. Another is chlorophenols, which is widely used as a preservative in leather, textiles, and wood industries because of their biocidal agent; it was reported to be toxic to the terrestrial ecosystem and can cause mutation. Persistent Organic Pollutants, popularly known as POPs, are organic compounds produced through human activities. They are difficult to degrade and are quickly accumulating in our food chain. These compounds were produced for industrial processes, such as coolants for paints and electrical transformers, sealants for plasticizers and woods, and as dielectric fluids. Their toxicity and accumulation in our food chain has posed a severe threat to our ecosystem.

One of the potent pollutants identified in industrial wastewaters is inorganic salts, which are usually used as preservatives and therapeutic agents. Ammonia is a product of an organic nitrogenous waste obtained after their decay; its presence indicates the existence of organic wastes. According to the survey, it is estimated that from all salts used as preservatives and therapeutic agents, ~60% are total chlorides which, when released along with the effluents, might affect aquatic plants and certain species of animals. Chlorides released with industrial effluents are measured in terms of total dissolved solids (TDS), which subsidize the salinity with discharged wastewater. Another inorganic class discharged with wastewater is cyanide ions, which has a strong binding capacity with metal ions and has been extensively used for metal cleaning and electroplating in metal processing industries. It has also been found as the primary pollutant in the wastewaters discharged from gas and coke oven industries, in the form of gas and coke scrubber. The combination of sulfate and sulfide compounds causes severe health hazards and destructive environmental impacts. Hydrogen sulfide gas, which is formed due to oxygen deficiency in the existence of sulfates and some organic materials, results in cellular anoxia or hypoxia by inhibiting cytochrome oxidation and other oxidative enzyme activity. Dyes that are released along with wastewaters are intricately linked with toxicity and appeal of the discharged wastewater due to its residual color. Since these dyes preserve their color and structural makeup upon exposure to soil, sunlight, and microorganisms, it reveals their high resistance capacity against microbial degradation. Most of the dyes released in wastewaters belong to the class of azo dyes—which, under anoxic conditions, voluntarily gets converted into hazardous aromatic amines.

The day by day increase in the establishment of industries has amplified the release of toxic heavy metals in the environment, which is now a matter of great concern. Their contamination mainly exists in the aquatic ecosystem, where industries such as tanneries, metal plating, alloy industries, smelting, radiator manufacturing, mining operations, etc., dump their heavy metal contaminated wastewater directly (Kadirvelu et al., 2001). Thus, industrial wastewaters should be treated before their discharge into the ecosystem.

# Processing and Chemical Pollutants in Industries

# 2

A key factor for the development of any country's economy is industrialization, but the wastes released are one of the major sources of worldwide environmental pollution. In terms of impact on the ecosystem, the chemical industries are of significance since the wastewaters generated from these industries contain toxic pollutants. The effluents released from industries such as tannery, textile, food, pulp and paper, distillery, pharmaceutical, oil refinery, etc., is of major concern since these consist of an array of organic and inorganic recalcitrant pollutants and toxic heavy metals. The wastes generated from industries consist of high biological oxygen demand (BOD), low solid suspension, acids, bases, heavy metals, and other toxic materials. These pollutants from different industries cause severe soil and water pollution once it reaches the environment, and several fatal diseases such as neurological disorders, cancer, delayed nervous response, mutagenic and teratogenic changes, etc., when it enters the human or animal food chain. For environmental safety, proper treatment of these industrial wastewaters is required before discharge in the environment. Some of the pollution-causing industrial wastewaters have been described below.

## 2.1 PAPER INDUSTRY

A challenge for our environment is the discharge of wastes from the pulp and paper industry (P&P), but on the other hand, it shows its positive side by utilizing renewable and photosynthetic resources. For the production of about one metric ton of paper, ~70 m$^3$ of wastewaters are released, and the quality of wastewater generally depends on the nature of raw material utilized, type of finishing product, and the amount of water reused during the process (Latorre et al., 2007). P&P Industry utilizes 70% of water during its processing. After the implementation of internal cleaning processes, the P&P industry has increased the internal water recirculation process to reduce its water consumption, which in turn saves capital and decreases the utilization of inadequate environmental resources. Over the past 20 years, P&P industries have reduced water consumption by nearly half, and a production of 95% paper per ton over the past 30 years (Blanco et al., 2004).

Pulp and Paper industries generate wastewaters formed by various class pollutants of complex mixtures of organic materials such as lignin, extractives, and degradative carbohydrate products, and solids. The main steps in paper productions are wood preparation, pulping, pulp washing, screening, paper machine, coating operation, and bleaching—in which polluted wastewaters are released into the environment (Savant et al., 2006; Ugurlu and Karaoglu, 2009). The quality of wastewater generated mostly depends upon the type of raw materials used during processing, the amount of water utilized, and the recirculation of the wastewaters generated (Pokhrel and Viraraghavan, 2004). The wastewaters released from P&P industries consist of high values of BOD, COD, and chlorinated chemicals—collectively known as absorbable organic halides (AOX). Since 1990, the emission of AOX content, which is directly proportional to chlorine consumption in the bleaching process, has been reduced up to 80%. The fraction of organic compounds that can be easily degraded from the effluent depends on the ratio of BOD to COD (McCubbin and Folke, 1993). Among the total organic materials produced in the effluent, the chemical pulping process has been reported to generate poor biodegradable organics to more than 40%. The industrial wastewaters, if released into a freshwater body without proper treatment, might cause adverse effect by depleting its dissolved oxygen, causing unacceptable changes in water color, temperature, turbidity, solid contents of the receiving freshwater bodies; as a consequence, it causes a toxic effect on fishes and other aquatic organisms. For the protection of the environment, satisfying legal requirements should be taken by the industries in removing harmful and toxic compounds from the generated wastewaters before releasing them into the environment (Kamali and Khodaparst, 2015). For example, the US government has established rules and regulations for the discharge of wastewaters from P&P industries, which provide significant inducement for the discharge of pollutants in reduced form in the wastewater.

# 2.1.1 Sources and Characteristics of Pulp and Paper Industry Wastewaters

The wastewaters emerging from P&P industries are highly variable, especially when comparing one pulp or paper making process to another. Maximum variations in effluent characteristics are observed during specific kinds of pulping, bleaching, or paper making operations and on the utilization of freshwater (Hossain and Ismail, 2015). Typical pulp and paper manufacturing processes that release contaminated wastewaters are discussed below.

## 2.1.1.1 Debarking

This is the first process in manufacturing, where the first load of contaminated water is generated from the soaking of logs and bark removal. The contamination level from debarking is low when compared with other operations, since only mechanical pressures are involved in removing the bark. It can easily be treated through electro-coagulation methods (Vepasalainen et al., 2011). Besides, the production of wastewater is reduced if dry debarking is allowed, and this process makes it possible to obtain more energy in a power boiler (BREF, 2015).

## 2.1.1.2 Mechanical Pulping

The fibers in the wood are separated by the mechanical process for obtaining virgin pulp, which is most often used in the production of high-circulation magazines and newsprint papers. The pulp is generated through a mechanical process requiring a high amount of energy per unit mass of pulp production—which results in soluble and particulate materials being released into the water stream. Mechanical pulping helps in the softening of the lignin between fibers, allowing full-length fibers to be preserved for a long time during the separation process—which is often carried out at a high temperature (i.e., thermomechanical pulping or TMP). It is assumed that more materials are released into the wastewater due to heating but does not have any literary support (Willfor et al., 2003). Hemicellulose components of TMP are converted into negatively charged carboxylate species through peroxide-bleaching of thermomechanical pulp (BCTMP), which contributes as a contaminant in the wastewater (Miao et al., 2013). The high yield of pulp also contributes to a low level of COD to the P&P industries wastewater.

## 2.1.1.3 Kraft Pulping

Kraft pulping operation produce highly contaminated wastewaters since this process can solubilize about 30–60% of the solid mass during bleaching of either wood-based or non-wood cellulosic pulps. After the kraft cooking process, the black liquid was rich in lignin byproducts along with alkali, sodium sulfate, soaps of resin acids and fatty acids, and other contaminants (Lehto and Alen, 2015). A high percentage of solubilizing materials are circulated back to the chemical recovery systems from alkaline pulping under ideal conditions. However, chemical recovery becomes complicated when a high amount of silica is contained in the fibers because it deposits in the equipment as an inorganic scale (Deniz et al., 2004). Also, the conventional bleaching technologies based on chlorine dioxide, sodium hypochlorite and other related chemicals generate highly toxic wastewaters, which become corrosive to the instrument used for chemical recovery and discourage the recovery of toxic chemicals from wastewaters, making it highly toxic with unusual odor and color that needs proper treatment (Tielbaard et al., 2002). These pollutants from pulp bleaching become exceedingly difficult to remove from wastewater, and often harm water bodies with slime and scum formation, toxicity to aquatic organisms, and thermal impacts (Garg and Tripathi, 2011).

## 2.1.1.4 Sulfite Pulping Process

Due to low strength property, sulfite pulps are produced less than kraft pulp. These sulfite processes may only be used by changing the pH and type of base used (ammonium, calcium, magnesium, or sodium) during processing—some of which are acid bisulfite, neutral sulfite, or magnetite. During the sulfite cooking process, lingo-sulfonates, sugars, and other substances are produced, which are further utilized as raw materials to produce various chemical yields (BREF, 2015).

## 2.1.1.5 Paper Recycling Operations

The variability in nature of paper materials used, their contamination during use and recovery, and the use of additives during bleaching, ink removing, and dispersing of fibers produces a wide range of pollutants during the recovery of fibers from recycled papers (Muhamad et al., 2012). Wastewaters with high organic dissolved loads of anionic characters are released during the processing.

## 2.1.1.6 Papermaking Operations

Paper machine produces cleanest process water in the plant, and excessive water production in paper machines is purified through filtration to be reused in the papermaking process. Furthermore, when high water quality is required, the used water is subjected to further treatment such as ultra-filtration (UF). The processing water in papermaking operations consists of a variety of additives together with mineral filler products such as clays, calcium carbonate, and titanium dioxide. In the fiber slurry sizing agents like alkenyl succinic anhydride, alkyl ketene dimer or rosin products are added in the form of a slurry. In the case of producing colored papers, dyes are used along with these compounds but in low amounts, where removal of dyes becomes the primary treatment because of its high visibility.

## 2.1.2 Recalcitrant Organic Pollutants in P&P Industry Wastewaters

A variety of recalcitrant compounds are present in pulp and paper mill wastewaters, such as chlorinated resin acids, chlorinated phenols, chlorinated hydrocarbons, dioxins, and lingo-sulfonic acids (Singh and Srivastava, 2014). In most cases, the toxicity of P&P mill wastewater is very low but is characterized by high COD (i.e., 1,000–7,000 mg/L), low biodegradability ratio (BOD/COD) from 0.02 to 0.07, and suspended solids of very moderate strength (i.e., 500–2,000 mg/L). Compounds with chlorine content are recalcitrant since they consist of uncommon chemical structures such as carbonchlorine bonds (Mounteer et al., 2007). Earlier, it has been reported that the organic materials in wastewaters with high molecular weight are more recalcitrant to biological treatment methods than of low molecular weight (Savant et al., 2006). The dark color of the wastewater and its toxicity is imparted by compounds such as diterpene alcohols, juvaniones, resin acids, dissolved lignin, and its degradation products—hemicelluloses, fatty acids, phenols and tannins (Chopra and Singh, 2012).

# 2.2 DISTILLERY INDUSTRY

One of the most polluting industries—whose 88% of the raw materials get converted into wastes—is distilleries. It is estimated that for every liter of production of alcohol, around 15 L of the spent wash is released in distilleries (Ravikumar et al., 2007). For the largest number of chemical industries, alcohol serves as a primary chemical, and high production is necessary to fulfill the demand. Presently, there are ~315 distilleries in India with a total capacity to produce 3,250 million liters of alcohol per year, with a production of 40.4 billion liters of effluent (Mohana et al., 2009). Most of the distillery industries collaborate with a sugar mill and utilize the by-product of sugar cane known as molasses as the starting material in producing alcohol (Chowdhary and Bharagava, 2019).

## 2.2.1 Process of Manufacturing and Generation of Wastewater

The main product of the distillery industry (i.e., alcohol) is produced through cellulosic materials from grains, sugarcane molasses, grapes, sugarcane juice, and barley malt. Alcohol productions in distilleries occur in four main steps—feed preparation, fermentation, distillation, and packaging. Fermentation can take place in batches or continuous mode in a broth, where diluted sugarcane molasses are inoculated with yeast, and a yield of 6–8% is produced. For alcohol production in continuous mode, cellulosic substances are first de-lignified into cellulose and hemicellulose, and then hydrolyzed by acids to break it into simpler sugars. These sugars are, then, fermented to produce carbon dioxide and ethanol in the presence of yeast. The alcohol produced is collected in the form of vapor from the fermentation solutions, through distillation under pressure. The removal of alcohol is assisted through the sprinkling of carbon dioxide gas produced throughout the fermenting solution (Satyawali and Balkirshnan, 2007). Later, carbon dioxide gas is captured and utilized in the production of other additional ethanol and essential chemicals.

## 2.2.2 Characterization of Wastewater Produced During Manufacturing

A huge amount of water is consumed in alcohol distilleries during the production of alcohol, and consequently, massive quantities of toxic wastewaters are released into the environment. The characteristics of wastewaters produced from spent wash are inconsistent and depend on the type of raw materials and phases utilized during the production of ethanol (Pant and Adholeya, 2007). The spent wash generated from distillery industries are dark brown in color with low pH (5.4–4.5), high temperature, BOD (40,000–50,000 mg/L) and COD (80,000–100,000 mg/L) (CPCB, 2003). The presence of high loads of organic materials such as melanoidin, proteins, lignin, reduced sugars, waxes, polysaccharides, etc., results in high values of

BOD and COD of the wastewater (Melamane et al., 2007). About 2% of melanoidins are present in the spent wash with a molecular weight between 5,000 and 40,000 Da, empirical formula of $C_{17-18}H_{26-27}O_{10}$-N, and antioxidant properties that make it toxic (Manisankar et al., 2004). Various technologies have opted for the treatment of these toxic spent washes but none of them have proved to be effective and economically useful to obtain the standard norms set by CPCB, India.

## 2.3 TEXTILE INDUSTRY

Industrialization has led to the development of a series of industries, including the textile industry, which is based on the utilization of synthetic dyes. Synthetic dyes are not only used in textile industries but are also extensively used in paper printing, color photography, and in food industries. Dyes have now become an essential part of our civilization, but are also responsible for creating environmental pollution, especially when released with the wastewaters generated from various textile mills and industries. Dyes are aromatic and heterocyclic compounds with variation in structures such as acid, azo, anthraquinone-based, basic, disperse, diazo, reactive, and metal complex—but these dyes are often recalcitrant compounds, toxic, and even carcinogenic in nature. The main problem is the lack of data regarding the dyes, which creates an issue when it comes to identification of their properties and characteristics. The aforementioned dyes have been classified based on their mode of dyeing or on structural moieties, which reflects little knowledge on evaluation based on environmental purposes.

Textile dyes containing industrial wastewaters are released in vast quantities daily in natural bodies of water worldwide. Soils and freshwater systems get contaminated with dyes when industries release dye-containing wastewaters through poor handling of spent effluent, the inefficiency of the dyeing process, and poor treatment of wastes. Among these dyes, anthraquinone-based dyes are found to be the most resistant to degradation and remain colored for an extended time because of their fused aromatic structures. Basic dyes have high color intensity, so it becomes complicated to decolorize from wastewater, while metal-based dyes lead to the release of toxic metals into water supplies and tend to be carcinogenic in nature. Disperse dyes have the capacity to bioaccumulate, and heavy metal ions are found to have high concentrations in both algae and higher plants such as wheat—which gets irritated by the textile wastewaters. The first contaminant to be acknowledged in wastewater is color; this should be removed from wastewater before their discharge into any freshwater body since these make them unpleasant. The colors in wastewater contribute to the significant fraction of BOD in wastewaters; thus, their removal is more important than the dissolved colorless organic substances.

## 2.3.1 Generation and Characteristics of Textile Wastewater

The characteristics of textile wastewater usually depend on the type of textile manufactured and the chemicals used during the processing. The major constituents of textile wastewater—which is a threat not only to the environment but also to human health—are chemicals, color, odor, high BOD, COD, total solids, and traces of some heavy metals such as arsenic, chromium, copper, and zinc. One of the critical factors for successful trading in textiles is the processing steps. First, fibers are prepared, transformed into yarn, and finally into fabrics subjected to various wet processing stages, where unfixed dyes get washed away. After the wet process, textile products are subjected to dry processes, where most of the solid wastes are generated. Each wet processing step has been described below.

### 2.3.1.1 Sizing and Desizing

Sizing acts as a defensive, protective material as it modifies the absorption and characteristics of substances. The sizing process improves resistance and reduces the risk of yarn breakage. The selection of sizing agents is made based on fabric types, cost-effectiveness, removal, environmental-friendliness, effluent treatments, etc. Sizing agents can be naturally occurring substances such as cellulosic derivatives, protein-based starch, starch, and its derivatives, etc., or synthetic agents such as polyacrylates, polyesters, PVA, etc.

The removal process of size materials from the yarn is known as desizing, which involves acids, enzymes, oxidative, or removal of water-soluble sizes (Chowdhary et al., 2019). After desizing, the textile wastewaters released have a pH of 4–5 with high BOD range (i.e., 300–450 ppm) (Magdum et al., 2013). Starch used during the sizing process can be degraded by $H_2O_2$ oxidation into $CO_2$ and $H_2O$, while enzyme desizing gets converted into ethanol—which is further utilized as energy, reducing BOD lead from textile effluent.

### 2.3.1.2 Scouring

Scouring is a chemical washing process carried out for removing certain impurities or any added dirt particle or soil from yarns or fibers through bridge scour, hydrodynamic scour, ice scour or tidal scour.

## 2.3.1.3 Bleaching

Natural substances present give a creamy color to the fabrics; to achieve white and bright fabrics, it is essential to remove this. The entire process of removing color is known as bleaching. Initially, bleaching was done by chlorine, succeeded by hypochlorite due to their disinfecting ability. Now, it has been replaced by hydrogen peroxide and per-acetic acid—with the advantage of providing intense sheen and causing less destruction to the yarn (Liang and Wang, 2015).

## 2.3.1.4 Mercerization

Mercerization is the process of improving the shine or luster of cotton fabrics by treating it with a strong caustic alkaline solution of 18–24% by weight. During this process, cotton fabrics are first dipped in high concentrations of the caustic alkaline solution. After getting completely absorbed, the swollen fabrics are placed into the water—providing stress conditions to remove the alkali solution, giving the fabrics a permanent silk-like shine. This process also helps the fabrics absorb an increased amount of dye, and improve reaction rate with various dyes, texture, and stability form and strength (Lee et al., 2014).

## 2.3.1.5 Dyeing and Printing

Dyeing is where fabrics or yarns are colored by treating them with a variety of dyes in controlled conditions (temperature and time). The dyes have either auxochrome group or chromophore groups. Textile products are dyed from dye solutions, and printing from the thick paste of dye helps prevent them from spreading. Both the dyeing and printing process consist of a variety of dyes that are eventually released in wastewater, making them highly visible.

## 2.3.1.6 Finishing

Considered as the last process in textile manufacturing, finishing involves conversion of woven or knitted cloth into usable material, adding qualities like anti-bacterial, UV protection, and waterproof. It is also the final process that contributes to water pollution.

The wastewaters released from textile mills after processing and cleaning consist of highly toxic organic residues with a mixture of synthetic and versatile dyes. It has been estimated that ~8000 L of wastewater are released to produce a kilogram of product. The BOD level is 25 kg/kg of product, and the COD level is 80 kg/kg of products for reactive and azo dyes. For other dyes, the BOD level is 6 kg/kg, COD level is 25 kg/kg, oil & grease is 30 kg/kg, and suspended solids are 6 kg/kg of the product. Toxic effluents of textiles consist of treated sludge, spent acids, and residue dyes of yellow and orange pigment, chrome and chrome oxide, green pigments, azo dyes, iron blue pigments, yellow zinc pigments, and molybdate orange pigments. Various conventional and non-conventional treatment methods are applied for treating the textile industries' wastewater. If discharged without proper treatment, excessive amounts of COD may cause toxicity to the aquatic life and elevated BOD might deplete the oxygen of the receiving water body. The high color intensity of the wastewater makes it unfit for downstream purposes. Hydrophilic and recalcitrant textile dyes quickly enter the hydrosphere and cause disturbance to the balanced ecosystem. A tiny amount of dye (i.e., 1 ppm) is highly visible and affects water transparency and gas solubility in rivers, lakes, and other receiving water bodies. Through the aquatic food chain, these dyes may enter the human body through consumption of contaminated seafoods, causing serious health hazards. Thus, the contaminated effluents must be treated before their discharge in nature for safety.

# 2.4 TANNERY INDUSTRY

The tannery industry, which utilizes a substantial quantity of chemicals during the process of transforming animal hides to produce leather, has been regarded as the most polluting industrial sector. In most countries, the chrome tanning process is utilized due to its excellent leather production and smooth operation (Chowdhary et al., 2017). Chrome tanning is a wet process that requires a large amount of water—90% of which will be released as an effluent. During transforming process, a broad quantity of chemicals—colored compounds, toxic metals, sodium chlorides, sulfates, a variety of organic and inorganic compounds, biologically oxidizable tanning materials, putrefying suspended materials, etc.—are used and released with the wastewaters (Chandra and Chaudhary, 2013). The presence of these massive pollutants in the tannery wastewaters damage the aquatic life of the water bodies and soil profile of the land receiving it.

In the tannery industry, the highest amount of water is consumed during pre-tanning processes, while post-tanning process also expends a liberal amount of water. In the tanning process, the most polluting stage is known as the soaking stage and contributes around 50–55% to the total pollution load. Secondarily is the limiting stage, where hair, skin, protein, and emulsified proteins are removed from the hides and are released with the wastewaters—which increases their total solid contents. Lastly is the tan-yard process, where delimbing and bating of various amounts of chemicals such as ammonium salts, calcium salts, sulfide, etc. makes the wastewater of slightly alkaline in nature. The effluents released during the chrome tanning and preserving process consists of chrome, chlorides, sodium bicarbonates, sulfates, sulfuric acids, and a high concentration of total solids. Among these large varieties of chemicals used during tanning processing, only ~20% of them are utilized and the rest are released as wastes. In the post-tanning process, the significant pollutants released during processing are chrome salts, dyestuff residues, fatliquoring agents, x systems, organic materials, and various other solvents used during degreasing and finishing. An estimate ~300–400 million tons of solvents, toxic sludge, heavy metals, and other wastes are being discharged with tannery effluents into the water bodies each year worldwide.

The improper handling of pesticides, tanning processing chemicals, and treated hides and skins of animals generates toxic and hazardous materials, which can affect human health. After processing, the final complex tannery effluent released consists of high loads of dissolved and suspended solids, organic and inorganic materials, organic ammonia, and nitrogen and retained high pH. The reduced processing practices—using unprocessed conventional tanning methods and non-implementation of controlled wastewater releasing rules and regulations—have further increased pollution rates and related problems. In most developing countries, it is tragic that there are no consistent estimates of the amount and types of toxic and hazardous wastes available, and in some cases, proper documentation is also unavailable. Tannery industries are job and revenue-generating sectors. However, pollutants such as heavy metals, chemicals, organic and inorganic materials, etc., are generated from these industries and are of significant concern because of unsafe soil and water disposal that lead to severe health hazards.

## 2.4.1 Chemicals Used in Tanning and Leather Production

Tannery industries are being specialized to produce leather skins from small animals such as calves, goats, and sheep, while hides are processed from the skin of large animals such as buffaloes, cows, and horses. In the tanning process, hides/skins are converted into stable and non-decomposable products such as leathers, which are further used for various purposes. Based on tanning reagents used, the tanning processes can be classified into chrome or vegetable tanning. For achieving different types of end products, various chemicals and procedures are involved in tanning, and the kind and total amount of wastes generated varies. A semi-soluble protein "collagen" is present in hides/skins of animals which are converted into highly durable commercial forms of leathers through tanning, by using large amounts of chemicals such as alkalis, acids, tannins, sulfates, chromium salts, surfactants, dyes, phenolics, auxiliaries, sulphonated oils, biocide, etc. These chemicals are not completely fixed and end up mixing in wastewater. During the tanning process, poor chromium salt (50–70%) uptake results in waste of materials, which results in ecological disturbance. Additionally, other chemicals such as sulfonated oils, acrylic resins, formaldehyde, melamine, naphthalene, and phenol are applied during tanning or retaining process to soften the leather. To avoid the usage of many hazardous chemicals during industrial processes, numerous regulations have been passed by the Integrated Pollution Prevention and Control Directive (96/61/EC 1996; 200/1/EC 2008). The Directive for European Regulatory Framework has made specific rules and regulations on chemicals regarding their registration, evaluation, authorization, and restriction to avoid leather-producing industries in using leather auxiliary and chemicals which are not included in the safety data sheets. Furthermore, the directive has also restricted the market and use of product preparations constituting >0.1% of nonylphenol (NP) or nonylethoxyphenol (NPE) in Europe (Lofrano et al., 2013). Additionally, industries have been instructed to label all products containing >0.5% of phthalate composition such as benzyl butyl phthalate, di-butyl phthalate, and diethyl hexyl phthalate, since these compounds have the potential to create reproductive toxicity. The usage of formaldehyde as well as o-phenyl phenol has been restricted in leather finishing because of their carcinogenic potentiality. Furthermore, the use of several azo dyes and inorganic compounds such as cadmium sulfate and lead chromate has been restricted due to higher toxicity.

## 2.4.2 Generation of Solid Wastes

Apart from liquid wastes, a large quantity of non-biodegradable sludge or tanned solid wastes containing chromium is also generated from tannery industries. The wastes have limited applications; thus, their disposal might cause serious environmental problems. Most of the available conventional treatments for solid wastes are not environmentally-viable because of the emission of nitrogen oxide, hydrogen cyanide, ammonia, and the transformation and leaching of Cr(III) into Cr(VI) from tannery wastes (Dixit et al., 2015). Therefore, the amalgamation of the aerobic with anaerobic treatment process might be a suitable option for tannery wastes treatment constituting all these toxic and recalcitrant hazardous chemicals. After treatment, the remaining wastes can be recycled and reused as a useful product or raw material.

# 2.5 PHARMACEUTICAL INDUSTRY

Pharmaceutical industries are one of the top-ranked science-based Indian industries which deal with the manufacturing of drugs. According to the draft national pharmaceutical policy 2006, the total market of Indian pharmaceuticals is 24,440 crores (Shah, 2007). The industry spends nearly 3% of its total sales on Research and Development (R&D) activities, but it is expected to increase to 5% in the coming years since R&D is the foundation of pharmaceutical industries. The corporate and multinational companies have their separate R&D facilities to furnish the research and follow new methods to satisfy their demands. Thus, the R&D section of pharmaceutical industries is emerging as a fast-growing industry. To develop a new drug, many cooperative efforts of trained employees specializing in different fields such as biochemistry, chemical engineering, organic and analytical chemistry, medicinal, microbiology, physiology, pharmacology, pathology, and toxicology are required. As a result of this diversity, an extensive range of biological as well as chemical wastes are produced in wastewaters, making it complicated to treat.

## 2.5.1 Characteristics of Wastewater Produced

Wastewater released from pharmaceutical industries has high concentrations of salts, organic materials, and microbial toxicity, increasing its non-biodegradability. Since pharmaceutical industries work based on batch mode processes, they utilize several types of raw materials during production, which causes variations in wastewaters with loads of toxic pollutants (Xin and Guoyi, 2015). Characteristics of wastewaters differ from one pharmaceutical industry to another. Biopharmaceutical industry wastewaters are known for varying quantities of high sodium concentration, low carbon/nitrogen (C/N) ratio, complicated composition, high sulfate concentrations, high chroma, and biological toxicity. In comparison, chemical pharmacy wastewater is non-biodegradable and has high salt concentration, causing toxicity to microbiota. The industries producing Chinese medicines have wastewaters that consist of alkali contents, cellulose, sugar, glycosides, tannins, anthraquinone, lignin, organic pigments, and some other organic materials (Yu, 2013).

# 2.6 OTHER INDUSTRIES

Apart from the different industries mentioned, there are other businesses that regularly release recalcitrant and toxic compounds, such as oil refinery industries, food industries, etc. Oil refinery industries generate wastes that are high in aromatic concentration, aliphatic petroleum hydrocarbons, etc., and loaded with a variety of toxic chemicals. The wastewater generated during crude oil extraction from oil wells has high COD and low biodegradability. Other recalcitrant organic pollutants that are produced are PAHs, polymers, benzenes, phenols, surfactants, radioactive substances, hummus, and different kinds of heavy mineral oils. If the effluents are discharged directly into a receiving body, it can cause toxic effects to aquatic life and to the body of water per se. Thus, oil refinery wastewater needs to be treated before their discharge into the environment.

Another essential industry is the food industry, which produces products that fulfill our daily health needs. The wastewaters generated from food processing also cause pollution due to its high COD and BOD content. As compared to other industrial sectors, food processing industries require a considerable amount of water throughout their operations—production, cleaning, sanitization, cooling, and material transport. Increased demand for food production involves a large amount of sludge as well as wastewater production and, consequently, the cost of treatment plants. The problem is that the wastewaters do not meet the standards set by the environmental regulations. Therefore, industries should treat released wastewater for sanitary purposes.

# Ecotoxicological and Health Implications

# 3

In modern society, chemicals are widely used in areas such as agriculture (e.g., pesticides), medicine (e.g., pharmaceuticals), cosmetic production, (e.g., powder, sunscreens) and mostly industrial sectors (e.g., acids, salts, solvents, coolants, etc.). In the European Union, ~33 million chemicals were commercially available in the year 2015—an estimated 100,000 of which are in use and over 1 ton of ~30,000 more chemicals are being produced annually (Breithaupt, 2006). These chemicals are released intentionally (spraying of pesticides) or unintentionally (grassing out or leaching into the environment), where they enter through different pathways depending on climatic, geological, hydrological or some other used patterns. These entry pathways of chemicals into our ecosystem might include:

1. The direct release of effluents from industries through different processing, mining, effluent treatment plants (ETPs), or through accidental spills;
2. Run-off water from subsurface flows or land surfaces frequently afterward drizzles;
3. Disposal or erosion of wastes from the surface, which might lead to desorption, diffusion of re-suspension of chemicals into the water level; and
4. Through atmospheric deposition.

According to survey, tons of industrial wastewaters are effluxed indiscriminately into lands, lagoons, rivers, and streams daily. The release of untreated or poorly treated industrial wastewaters constituting nutrients, toxic heavy metals, non-biodegradable organic and inorganic materials, and other toxicants deteriorate these receiving freshwater systems. Industrial wastewaters/effluents are the liquid wastes produced from various industrial activities. Over the years, the inappropriate disposal of these liquid wastes into the environment has become a major concern to industrialists as well as the government. In many cases, the industrial wastewaters do not meet the standards of these processes because of the application of prohibited toxic chemical pollutants in industries which remain even after pre-treatment methods. Consequently, high loads of toxic and recalcitrant chemical pollutants accumulate in the environment, causing ecosystem pollution, and producing severe health hazards. Therefore, there is a need for effective treatment of effluents from several industries before their discharge into a public water body. The ecological toxicity as well as health hazards caused by these toxic pollutants are described below.

# 3.1 ECOTOXICITY

With the advances in scientific knowledge, the rate of pollution can be controlled by measuring environmental contaminations. As knowledge on the environmental impacts of wastewater and the drawbacks of sophisticated conventional methods increases, the utilization of advanced treatment methods has become more common. Industrial effluents/wastewaters released into the environment after poor treatment have a toxic effect on the water bodies receiving them, as described in Figure 3.1. The toxic effects may be acute or cumulative. The acute toxic effects by industrial wastewaters are created by high concentrations of chlorine, ammonia, demanding oxygen materials, toxic heavy metals, inorganic, and recalcitrant organic pollutants. In comparison, cumulative effects are caused by accumulation of toxic pollutants through industrial wastewaters in receiving water bodies, which becomes noticeable only after a certain level (Chambers et al., 1997). For optimum function and survival, aquatic organisms have a range of temperatures, and a sudden change in these can reduce or intimidate their reproductive cycle, growth, and life. The industrial wastewaters released into freshwater bodies after treatment are full of organic loads, which may add to the oxygen demand level of the receiving body. Furthermore, when a freshwater body receives an ill-treated industrial wastewater, it results in increased depletion of the dissolved oxygen (DO), and its level below 5 mg/L adversely affect the aquatic ecosystem. The proper concentration of oxygen in the aquatic ecosystem is essential in maintaining the biological life; if wastewater is poorly treated, it affects the aquatic flora and fauna of receiving system. The concentration of dissolved oxygen below 5 mg/L can cause a negative effect on aquatic organisms of the water receiving wastewater. The concentration of dissolved oxygen has been reported to be between 4.15–6.26 mg/L

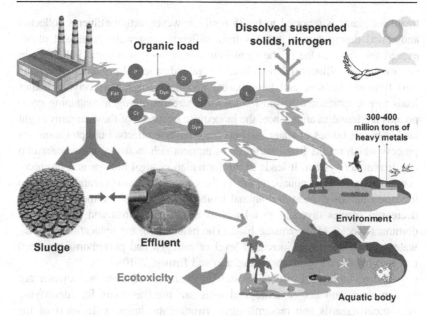

**FIGURE 3.1**   An overview of environmental pollutants and its toxicity.

during autumn, 4.96–6.69 mg/L during spring, 4.99–5.38 mg/L during summer, and 4.85–11.22 mg/L during winter, which proves that seasons have a significant influence on the DO level in the water body (Igbinosa and Okoh, 2009).

Compared to surface water, the low level of DO in industrial wastewater is due to the presence of degradable organic compounds. A low level of DO in water leads to impairment in some species and can eventually lead to their death. The estimation of organic pollution load in water and wastewater is usually done by measuring the range of Biological Oxygen Demand (BOD) and Chemical Oxygen Demand (COD)—which are the essential parameters in checking wastewater treatment plant efficiency and their facilities. The low-level values of BOD and COD is expected in surface water, which is necessary for life sustenance in an aquatic ecosystem, as elevated levels of BOD and COD harm aquatic life, especially fishes. In river systems, the low level of BOD and COD indicates decent quality of water, while high values of BOD and COD signifies polluted water. The BOD-COD and DO concentrations in water have an inverse relationship. DO is mostly consumed by bacteria when large loads of biodegradable organic materials are present in water. In the case of industrial wastewater, the threshold drop of the DO level has a negative impact on aquatic life (affecting fish and other life forms), rendering their life-sustaining functions, such as growth and reproduction, useless. The range of COD in wastewaters from several treatment plants is reported to be 75 mg/L; however, actual effluents collected and tested during several months from different wastewater treatment plants exceed this figure. One of the significant contributors of organic pollutants in surface water is effluents released from several industries. The addition of various ions (nitrates, nitrates, and phosphorus) into the wastewater-receiving bodies leads to eutrophication. In most wastewater streams, nitrogen-containing compounds are found in abundance; the inadequate treatment of these streams might lead to bigger bodies of water and can cause adverse effects. Eutrophication is a process which results from the influx of nutrient-rich industrial wastewater into any freshwater system. It leads to the formation of algal blooms and promotes continuous growth of aquatic plants in the ecosystem. Eutrophication results in increased turbidity, plant and animal biomass, and rate of sedimentation, with decreased species diversity that leads to anoxic conditions and modifies the dominant species of the aquatic biota. The induction of eutrophication in freshwater system due to an increased level of nitrogen and phosphorus has been reported by several researchers (Lofrano and Brown, 2010).

Today, biological effects caused by industrial effluents/wastewater are fundamental, and eco-toxicological tests are used as tools for identifying ecological hazards and recognizing environmental impacts. In most of the countries, ecotoxicity tests are used for the management of industrial wastewaters; they play a significant role in direct toxicity assessment as support in making decisions on a regulatory or voluntary basis. For the surveillance of industrial wastewater, bioassay tests are also done (Power and Boumphrey, 2004). In the case of complex wastewaters, global evaluation should be done—which includes eco-toxicological tests to complement the chemical characterization of industrial effluents. This approach will help protect the biological treatment plants from toxic and hazardous influents, monitor the efficacy of wastewater treatment plants (WWTP), and evaluate the impacts of wastewaters (Gartiser et al., 2010a). For the assessment of complex organic materials and their mixtures through eco-toxicological tests, bioassays are the most suitable tool. Physico-chemical parameters alone are not enough to collect reliable information regarding treated wastewaters; therefore, toxicity tests must be combined with routine chemical analysis.

## 3.2 HEALTH HAZARDS

Serious health hazards are caused by the environmental pollutions from industrial wastewaters released into our ecosystem. It affects land and water, including their biotic and abiotic components. Industrial wastewater containing organic and inorganic complex compounds that are thrown into our ecosystem contribute a lot of toxic and hazardous pollutants. These toxic pollutants are released from chemical, food processing, leather tanning, oil, refining, paper and pulp, paint, plastic, pharmaceutical, pesticide, metal smelting, iron and steel, and textile industries. The rapid establishment of industries in developing countries increases waste effluents, causing major chaos to the ecology, environment, agriculture, aquaculture, and public health. One-third of the total water pollution in India has been reported to be from industrial wastewater discharges composed of solid and other hazardous wastes, which are of potential danger to our natural water systems. High concentrations of various heavy metals such as cadmium, copper, chromium, nickel, lead, etc., along with several organic and inorganic compounds, are also found in the industrial wastewaters, and are highly poisonous to various forms of life in the ecosystem.

Health hazards are associated in two ways. First, with health and safety problems of those who are working on the field or residing near the area where the industrial wastewaters are released. Second is through the utilization of contaminated products obtained from the use of wastewater, which consequently harms humans as well as animals through handling or consumption by secondary contamination (WHO, 2009). Therefore, random utilization of toxic industrial wastewaters to agricultural fields is one of the major global concerns, since the toxic compounds present in wastewater cannot be easily broken down into non-toxic forms, thus persisting in the environment causing a long-lasting effect on the ecosystem. The toxic metals—mostly heavy metals—present in industrial effluents are carcinogenic, cytotoxic, and mutagenic. Firm ground and surface water pollution cause severe health hazards to nearby surroundings; ruined soil fertility kills fishes as well as aquatic lives (Dey and Islam, 2015). Industries such as distilleries, refineries, textiles, and tanneries, etc. are chemical processing industries which utilize a tremendous amount of water at different processing stages and eventually release massive quantity of untreated or poorly treated wastewater and sludge directly into rivers and other freshwater bodies.

The biological degradation of the receiving water bodies depends on the quality of the industrial wastewater (i.e., the volume of effluents, chemical, and microbiological compositions/concentrations of the effluents released into the receiving water system). High concentrations of toxic pollutants, primarily organic materials of wastewater, boost BOD, COD, TDS, TSS, DO, etc., of the receiving freshwater body, making it unsuitable for drinking, irrigation, and other purposes. The high concentration of arsenic and chromium in drinking water causes cancer—particularly, skin cancer—as well as skin lesions like hyperkeratosis, and causes pigmentation problems. Occupational exposure through inhalation leads to lung cancer. The organic compounds used in several industrial processes are produced in wastewaters, which are toxic and non-acceptable to direct biological treatment. Thus, these wastewaters must be treated well to meet the discharging or recycling standards (Luan et al., 2012).

In most developing countries, industrial wastewaters are released into the sewage system. They are potentially utilized for irrigation in agricultural fields for fodder crops near the sewage disposal areas and can directly or indirectly be consumed by humans. Industrial wastewaters and sewage waters contaminate the agricultural soil by affecting both the soil health and its crop yield. The utilization of industrial wastewater for irrigation purposes on a regular basis results in poor quality of the soil, and gathering of toxic heavy metals into the soil may cause severe human and animal health threat (Kharche et al., 2011). The accumulation of toxic heavy metals in the soil changes its physico-chemical properties, making it inapt for further irrigation purposes. The toxic and hazardous pollutants seep into the soil profile, reaching groundwater level. After daily consumption, it may cause serious health problems in humans as well as livestock. The rate of seed germination, as well as germination speed percentage, is also affected by the industrial wastewaters in various crops such as *Vigna vulgaris*, *Vigna cylindrical,* and *Sorghum cermumas* due to the presence of organic and inorganic contents with acidic concentrations (Doke et al., 2011). With the increased use of industrial wastewaters for irrigation, growth parameters of crop such as radical and plumule length, their fresh and dry weight, carotenoid and chlorophyll content, and gradual decline in root and seedling length are also affected. The high salt concentration of soil also affects the growth rate of plants, high salinity and dissolved salts increases the osmotic pressure resulting in decreased availability of water to plants and to their retarded growth.

Pollutants such as chromium, tannins, chlorides, sulfides, sulfates, organic chemicals; synthetic chemicals such as pesticides (pentachlorophenol), dyes, finishing agents, chemical solvents, etc., are associated with industrial wastewaters. These are not completely absorbed during processing and the majority are released into the environment without adequate treatment, causing skin and blood infections upon direct contact. The eyes and respiratory system are mostly affected upon exposure to toxic chemicals and pesticides. Exposure to toxic chemical dust and hazardous compounds leads to intestinal infections and chronic respiratory disorders. Contact with a small quantity of chloride and hazardous phenolic compounds cause chemical burns and poisoning. These results show these compounds are toxic to humans and animals, whether in small or large degrees. It is alarming, since these can cause not only acute toxicity, but also genotoxic and mutagenic effects. After being released into the ground or other water bodies, these toxic chemicals get accumulated into the food chain and directly affect human as well as other living organisms (Nadal et al., 2004). The chemical pollutants may enter the human body through inhalation, ingestion, or by dermal absorption, which can create local organ defects (e.g., skin, lungs, or gastric system), and can also produce a systemic effect by damaging the cardiovascular system, digestive system, urinary system, immune system, reproductive system, and nervous system through the absorption or circulation of pollutants in the blood and its distribution to the whole body. The carcinogenic, mutagenic, or teratogenic effects of chemical pollutants on humans depend on the nature and level of exposure.

The degree to which any hazardous effect is shown in the human body is defined as toxicity, which is resolved by studying the interactions between the body and chemical pollutant dose entering. Some pollutants produce a harmful effect at specific doses and can even be beneficial at low doses, and this is determined through the dose-response curve relationship. The assessment of the risk of exposure to human health is derived through toxicological reference values, defined as the human toxicological risk limits or human criteria values. The toxicological reference values are reviewed from the toxicological data obtained from animal studies, environmental and occupational epidemiological studies, and from the scientific mechanisms of absorption, metabolism, transport, and toxicity of pollutants within the human body. By reviewing the toxicity data, the critical health effects and target endpoints can be determined by evaluating the potentiality of the chemical pollutants to create adverse effects on human health and its exposure conditions which damages human health. It also helps in identifying chemical causes and target organs or systems that may get damaged; data is collected based on intakes from air, food, water, and other relevant sources (Burdon et al., 2016).

# 3.3 REMEDY

The deposition of chemical pollutants in the environment should be under surveillance to avoid detrimental and hazardous effects upon exposure. Its remedy should be defined upon cleaning up of the contaminated sites. Several analytical methods such as gas chromatography/mass spectrometry (GC/MS) are available, which are sensitive and specific in identifying and quantifying the chemical compositions on environmental conditions, and their complexity associated with structures. These analytical methods, however, are to be operated on a regular and rapid basis and require online environmental and bioremediation process monitoring and control. To overcome this, whole living cell microorganisms have been found to indicate the presence of deleterious chemical pollutants through signals in response to the exposure of targeted chemicals measurable. This method has been utilized under the monitoring and treatment of plentiful environmental hazards creating chemical pollutants.

# Treatment Technologies for Industrial Wastewater

# 4

Adequate and cost-effective treatment of wastewater is a more challenging task. Indeed, some of the industrial processing schemes haven't been implemented because of their excessive costs and difficulties allied with the treatment of the wastewaters generated from industries. In most countries, large-scale environmental initiatives have been taken, which resulted in the application of strict rules and regulations regarding the discharge of industrial wastewaters into the environment. To meet the standards, industrial wastewater systems need expensive upgraded programs, but some industries could not even reach those modified limitations.

The wastewaters discharged from industries usually consist of a wide range of substances that can't be reduced easily, though they are passed from various treatment stages for their separation. The first step—primary treatment—includes basic physical methods for the separation of solids, large particles, and oils through screeners, primary clarifiers, and oil separators. The next step—secondary treatment—is where suspended and residual organic compounds are broken through biological agents; this treatment process is regarded as the core of the treatment unit. One of the simplest, most cost-effective, and high-performing treatment methods known is the aerated activated sludge treatment process. This treatment process includes the anaerobic and aerobic processes, which increases its efficiency in removing various soluble, biodegradable organic pollutants. Because of the rigid treatment regulations, the use of chemical oxidation and membrane-based techniques has increased for the treatment of industrial wastewaters. The last step is the tertiary treatment process, which is considered as the polishing and finishing stage in the process of treating wastewater. This step uses activated carbon filters during treatment. This chapter will highlight the recent and most efficient treatment technologies, all will be discussed below.

# 4.1 CONVENTIONAL TREATMENT APPROACHES

A combination of physical, chemical, and biological processes is included in the conventional wastewater treatment processes, which are not only operated to remove solids and organic materials but also nutrients from the wastewaters. In endless ways, we can say that conventional treatment processes include different degrees of treatment levels for wastewater—preliminary, primary, secondary, and tertiary treatments. In most countries, the last or tertiary treatment step includes disinfectants for removing pathogens from wastewater. All these conventional wastewater treatment steps have been discussed below.

## 4.1.1 Preliminary Treatments

The aim of the preliminary treatment is the removal of massive and granular solids usually found in wastewater through various treatment operations—grit removal, coarse screening, and sometimes, comminuting particles. Comminuting the large particles helps in their removal (in the form of sludge) in continuous treatment processes. For smooth removal of these solid granules from the wastewater, it is important to enhance the operation as well as maintenance of the treatment units. To prevent the settling of organic materials, the high-velocity water or air is sustained through the grit chambers, which are maintained through flow measurement devices. In most of the wastewater treatment plants, the grit chamber method is not included as a preliminary treatment step.

## 4.1.2 Primary Treatment

After preliminary treatment, the wastewaters are subjected to primary treatment processes, where settleable organic and inorganic solids are removed through sedimentation and floating materials are removed by gliding. During this step, ~50–70% of TSS (total suspended solids), 65% of oil and grease, and 25–50% of BOD (Biochemical oxygen demand) is removed. In the primary sedimentation separation process, some organic nitrogen, phosphorus, and heavy metals are removed, except for colloidal and dissolved constituents. The effluents discharged from the sedimentation units are referred to as primary effluent. The primary treatment has been regarded as the minimum level of pre-application treatment in most industrialized countries for the treatment of wastewaters used for irrigation purposes. If wastewaters are used for irrigating crops rather than human consumption, then it should be treated efficiently. To prevent any inconvenience in flow-equalizing or storing reservoirs, the wastewaters should be treated even though they are not utilized for irrigation purposes.

The basins of the primary sedimentation tanks are kept either circular or rectangular, typically with a depth of 3–5 cm with a hydraulic retention time between 2–3 hours. Preliminary solids settled at the bottom of the tanks are removed through sludge rakes, which fix the sludge to the central well and from there, it is pumped to sludge processing units. The primary sludge in large sewage treatment plants is biologically processed through anaerobic digestions, where both anaerobic and facultative bacteria break down the organic materials into sludge—which reduces the disposal volume and improves their characteristics. The process of anaerobic digestion is carried out in a 7–14 m deep in a covered tank for about ten days for high rate digestion and up to 60 or more days in standard digesters. The gas—methane—produced during the digestion process is recovered as a source of energy. The sludge produced from sewage treatment plants is directly applied in process storage and to the lands.

## 4.1.3 Secondary Treatment

After the primary treatment, the effluents are further subjected to secondary treatment for the removal of remaining organic residuals and suspended solids. In most cases, secondary treatments are followed by the primary treatments involving the removal of biodegradable organic materials by using aerobic treatment processes. Aerobic biological treatment processes metabolize the organic materials present in the wastewaters by producing more microorganisms and some inorganic byproducts such as $CO_2$, $H_2O$, and $NH_3$. Several aerobic biological methods are used in the secondary treatment processes based on the oxygen utilization by the microorganisms and the metabolization rate of the organic materials.

After treatment processes, microorganisms should be separated from the treated effluents through the sedimentation process to produce simplified secondary effluents. The biological sludge recovered during secondary treatments is combined with the primary sludge for further sludge processing. The high-rate processes involved in secondary treatments include trickling filters, activated sludge, oxidation ditches, and rotating biological contactors, which are described below.

### 4.1.3.1 Trickling Filters

In general, a trickling filter is a filter that consists of a basin or tower that is filled with supporting media—plastic shapes, stones, or wooden slats—where effluents are applied erratically or sometimes unremittingly. The microorganisms get attached on the surface of the supporting media, forming a biological film or layer where organic materials get metabolized by diffusing into the film. Oxygen is regularly supplied onto the biofilm layer through natural up or down the flow of air, depending on the relative temperature of the effluents being treated. As the new microorganisms grow, the thickness of the biofilm increases, which should be disposed periodically. The biofilm slops should be separated from the secondary clarifiers and discharged to sludge. Remaining liquids are regarded as secondary effluents.

### 4.1.3.2 Activated Sludge

In an activated sludge process, an aeration tank consisting of effluents and microorganisms are utilized and vigorously mixed through aeration devices, commonly including submerged diffusers which help supply oxygen to the microorganisms. To obtain the clarified secondary effluent, the microorganisms are separated (through sedimentation) from the liquid effluent following the aeration steps. To maintain a higher level of mixed liquor suspended solids in the aeration tanks, a portion of biological sludge is regularly recycled, and the rest are subjected to sludge processing to maintain a constant concentration of microorganisms in the system. Several other processes, such as oxidation ponds and extended aerations, are in widespread use and are identical to the basic activated sludge process with little variations.

### 4.1.3.3 Rotating Biological Contactors (RBCs)

These are fixed-film reactors like bio-filters where microorganisms attach to the supporting media. In this treatment process, the support media consists of various slowly rotating discs partially submerged in the reactor containing the wastewater. Oxygen is supplied to the microorganisms attached to the support media by the turbulence from the rotation of the discs. Typically, 85% of the $BOD_5$ and suspended solids, along with some heavy metals, are removed initially from the raw effluents in this high-rate biological treatment process. The effluents generated from this are of a slightly low quality than the effluents released from activated sludge. When the effluent released from RBCs is disinfected, a substantial number of microorganisms remain; only a little amount of nitrogen, organic compounds, phosphorus, non-biodegradable, or dissolved minerals are removed.

## 4.1.4 Tertiary Treatment

Tertiary treatment, more commonly known as advance wastewater treatment, removes specific wastewater constituents that were not removed by secondary treatment processes. Since advanced treatment methods (i.e., tertiary treatments) usually follow high-rate secondary treatment processes, individual treatment processes become necessary for the removal of additional suspended solids, dissolved solids, nitrogen, phosphorus, heavy metals, and organic materials. However, these advanced treatment techniques are sometimes used in place of secondary treatments or are combined with primary or secondary treatment methods. The wastewater from the primary clarifiers is flown to the reactors, which is separated into five zones—the first zone is meant to condition the group of bacteria responsible for the removal of phosphorus by adding stress under low oxidation-reduction conditions and rests for nitrogen gas removal.

These biological treatment methods cost more than the activated sludge process. Additionally, these methods are regarded can be complex for developing countries as they require skilled operations to achieve consistent results. In most situations where the probability of risk to human exposure is high, the primary intention of the treatment is to reduce the enteric viruses or other pathogenic microorganisms. Viruses are reserved by suspended and colloidal solids in the water; for effective disinfection, these solids should be removed through advanced treatment before disinfection. Secondary treatment—when followed by chemical coagulation, sedimentation, filtration, and disinfection—produces a detectable virus-free effluent with the last step of ozonation treatment.

# New Technologies Used in Wastewater Treatment 5

Conventional wastewater treatment technologies have been used worldwide to remove the toxic pollutants and microbial contaminants present in wastewater, which has been a source of concern to the environment and public health. Over the last two decades, the efficacy of these processes has been limited because of two new challenges (Mallevialle et al., 1996).

- The first challenge is the availability of fresh and quality water to the public. Wastewater-releasing sectors have been required to adhere to rules regarding the regulation of maximum contaminant levels (MCLs) in their sectors due to public concern regarding pollution and safety. Exacting standards have been set over the range of contaminants—nitrogen, phosphorus, sulfur, etc., and synthetic organic and inorganic compounds—because of their adverse effect on humans as well as the environment.
- The second challenge is the rapid industrialization and population growth that contribute to the decrease in freshwater sources.

The treatment of wastewater is particularly important, but the recovery of pollutants used during different processes and reusing of treated wastewater has also become critical. This creates more problems to the arid or semi-arid areas where the supply of freshwater—including irrigational water—is a prohibitive cost. The growing concern regarding the release of more toxic and recalcitrant compounds contaminating the freshwater sources is now justifying the reclamation of the toxic wastewaters being released. Thus, advanced treatment technologies have been utilized to remove toxic pollutants that remained after conventional treatment technologies. The development of advanced treatment processes has improved in versatility and costs of these processes at an industrial scale. In a comparative study, it was determined that the cost of a new membrane filtration plant was at par with conventional treatment processes with a bulk of 20,000 $m^3$/day (Wiesner et al., 1994). To utilize economic resources responsibly and resolve new challenges from conventional treatment equipment, several new treatment technologies—advance oxidation processes (AOPs), membrane filtration methods, and other green technologies like phytoremediation, bioremediation, algal treatment, etc.—have been proven to successfully remove a range of toxic contaminants from wastewaters.

---

# 5.1 REVERSE OSMOSIS

---

In arid and highly populated regions of the world, the industrial wastewater/effluent recovered through different treatment processes has become a sustainable means of supplementing water. According to literary survey, the stumpy quality of the wastewater after their treatment, limited its reuse but their quality can be improved through a variety of treatment technologies. During the treatment processes of wastewater, removal of dissolved ions and other organic materials has been the most difficult. Reverse osmosis (RO) treatment has been proven to be the most effective method to remove dissolved and organic materials; however, they might encounter operational issues due to the repugnant smell of the wastewater. These issues, if not treated properly, might stain RO membranes and lead to its frequent cleaning, increased plant downtime, high operating pressures, and shorter membrane life. After improving the process conditions and membrane products, a success has been reported by using RO membranes that result in less odor (Kochany, 2007).

Reverse osmosis technology has been recognized as a successful process for removing salts and other impurities fromwastewater—improving its quality and restoring its reusability. Other benefits include reduced purchases, reduced discharge, and conservation of water resources. Reverse osmosis units are often a combination of the mechanical filter with an activated carbon filter. In this process, effluents first pass through a mechanical filter that removes sand and large particles. Then, they pass through a reverse osmosis unit, and lastly through an activated carbon filter to remove organic compounds. Wastewater is passed through a semipermeable membrane in the reverse osmosis process, which helps reduce inorganic materials such as sulfate, calcium, magnesium, potassium, radium, nitrate, sodium, phosphorus, fluoride, and some organic matters such as pesticides. Drinking water contaminated with naturally occurring arsenic has now become a very decisive problem in many parts of the world (Hare et al., 2017, 2018, 2019), so RO membranes are used to remove arsenic metal, which occurs naturally and contaminates drinking water through rock and mineral erosion, or due to human activities like coal burning, paper production, mining, and cement manufacturing.

## 5.2 MEMBRANE TREATMENT

One of the recognized key technologies for the separation of pollutants is membrane technology. Membranes used in this technology act as selective barriers—driven by any pressure gradient and chemical or electrical potential across the membranes—which separate two distinct phases, only permitting specific components. Since membrane technologies depend on physical separation without the addition of any chemical, they are the best alternative to conventional wastewater treatments such as coagulation, distillation, precipitation, ion exchange, etc. (Mishra et al., 2019). The main appeal of this membrane technology process that makes it different is its less energy consumption, less processing steps, great split-up tendency, and higher quality of end product; however, their conflict to chemical, mechanical, and thermal effects limits application. Innovations and improvements regarding chemical and morphological designs of membrane materials—their element and module designing, anti-fouling membranes, etc.—are needed.

Recently, three generic membrane bioreactors (MBRs) have been developed—a combination of membrane technology and biological reactors—for the treatment of wastewaters. The aim of this generic bioreactor is easy separation and retention of solids, good aeration without bubbles, and organic pollutants extraction from effluents. The membranes are used as a biological process for separating and retaining the biomass in the reactors. An increase in water consumption demand and their necessity have demonstrated the treatment processes related to effluents (Boman et al., 1991). From this point of view, the membrane filtration process offers immense potential applications in the treatment of a variety of industrial wastewaters, as described in Table 5.1. These processes are pressure-driven—capable of clarification, concentration, and separation of organic matters from effluents. Some of the most common membrane filtration types are:

**TABLE 5.1**   Application of membrane filtration in wastewater treatment

| Membrane filtration | Wastewater source | Alignment | Consequential effects |
|---|---|---|---|
| Ultrafiltration (UF) | Pulp mill effluents | Tubular | Helps in removing COD, AOX, and toxicity up to 55–60%, 65–75%, and 50% respectively which is >98.9% for removal of COD, AOX and $Cl^-$ with a combination of UF-RO |
| | Paper machine white paper | Compact tubular, vibratory, high shear rotary | Helps in producing water quality which is suitable for internal recycling; by adjusting the pH pretreatments can be done and fixative addition increases the flux by 20% |
| | Oil and grease waste | Dead-end flats sheet; high shear rotary | Helps in removing >97% of both oil & grease and suspended solids |
| | Brewery wastewater | Hollow fiber | Efficiently removes 82% of COD at the rate of 2 kg COD ($m^3$ d) |
| Microfiltration (MF) | Paper machine white paper | Compact tubular, vibratory, high shear rotary | Helps in producing water quality which is suitable for internal recycling; by adjusting the pH pretreatments can be done and fixative addition increases the flux by 20% |
| Nano-filtration (NF) | Papermill effluents | Flat sheet test cell | Helps in rejecting >98% of both TOC and color efficiently but results in 50% declination of flux at |

| Membrane filtration | Wastewater source | Alignment | Consequential effects |
|---|---|---|---|
| | | | the rate of 89% of water recovery |
| | Paper machine white paper | Compact tubular, vibratory, high shear rotary | Helps in producing water quality which is suitable for internal recycling; by adjusting the pH pretreatments can be done and fixative addition increases the flux by 20% |
| | Textile wastewater | Tubular | Helps in removing >99% of both color & copper and 85% of salt at a rate of 85% of water recovery |

## 5.2.1 Micro-Filtration

Micro-filtration is a pretreatment process for reverse osmosis or nano-filtration, used to separate suspended solids; colloid particles form industrial effluents or macromolecules greater than the filtration size of 0.1–1 μm. This type of filtration process is used in dye baths of textile industries to separate dye pigments. Filters used in micro-filtration techniques are made up of specific polymers such as polycarbonate, polypropylene, polysulfone, polyether sulfone, polyvinylidene difluoride, polyvinylidene fluoride, polytetrafluoroethylene, etc. Whenever hot temperature or extraordinary chemical resistance operation is required during the treatment process, alumina, carbon, ceramic, glass, sintered metal, or zirconia-coated carbon membranes are employed in the micro-filtration technique.

## 5.2.2 Ultra-Filtration

Like micro-filtration, it is a pretreatment process for reverse osmosis and can be used in combination with biological reactors to remove heavy metal oxides of 1 ppm or less. This process is mostly used for separating macromolecules and other pollutants such as dyes used in textile industries, but their elimination is only 31–76%. The main drawback of this process is that quality of the effluent after treatment does not allow its reuse for sensitive processes, and only 40% of the recycled wastewater can be used in stages where salinity is not a problem. The membranes used in this process are made up of polymeric substances such as acrylic copolymers, nylon-6, polypropylene, polysulfone, polytetrafluoroethylene, polyvinyl chlorides, etc.

## 5.2.3 Nano-Filtration

Nano-filtration is a process that is used in combination with adsorption to reduce the polarization concentration during the treatment process. Nano-filtration membranes are tremendously sensitive to odor created by macromolecules and colloidal substances. The nano-filtration membranes are mostly composed of acetate and aromatic polyamides, which retain divalent ions, dyeing auxiliaries, hydrolyzed reactive dyes, large monovalent dyes, and low-molecular-weight organic compounds. Apart from these materials, the nano-filtration membranes are also made up of some inorganic materials such as carbon-based membranes, ceramics, zirconia, etc. According to survey, the typical nano-filtration flux rate is 5–30 gross flow per day. Approximately 90% of color removal rate has been reported through treatment with a single nano-filtration process in textile effluents, and in the case of other effluents, a combination with micro-filtration was found to be a useful treatment process. The main drawback of this process is the accumulation of the dissolved solids, making discharge of treated effluents in channels almost impossible. The nano-filtration treatment process has been satisfactory in the textile wastewaters decolorization method.

# 5.3 OXIDATION PROCESS

The process where electron is transferred from one constituent to another is known as the oxidation process—it leads to a potential that helps other compounds obtain oxidation potentials. In terms of meeting with treated effluent legislation, chemical oxidation has appeared to be an appropriate elucidation that is used after the secondary treatment process for the destruction of non-biodegradable components. Chemical oxygen demand

(COD) is used as a reference parameter in the chemical oxidation treatment process. Effluent with smaller COD content can be treated easier than those with higher COD contents, since it requires the ingestion of extreme amounts of costly reactants. The chemical oxidation processes have been divided into the following two types:

1. Classical chemical process
2. Advanced oxidation processes (AOPs)

Solvents are not an integral part of any chemical compounds undergoing reactions; formerly, they play an essential role in synthesis and production. Solvents are extensively used in the classical chemical process to dissolve reactants, separate mixtures, extract and wash products, clean reaction gadgets, and scatter products for normal applications. Though the invention of organic solvents has led to remarkable advances in chemistry, the legacy has resulted in various environmental and health concern.

Advanced oxidation processes (AOPs) involve the generation of extremely volatile radicals—usually hydroxyl radicals—to purify wastewaters in sufficient quantities at ambient temperature and pressure. AOPs are the most favorable method of treatment for contaminated wastewater, surface, and groundwater consisting of non-biodegradable organic pollutants. Most of the organic compounds are attacked by the extraordinary highly reactive hydroxyl radical species.

These processes are unbelievably cheap, more efficient, and eco-friendly in biodegradation of toxic pollutants generated with wastewater. These toxic pollutants are degraded by hydroxyl radicals into harmless products. However, they also face technical and economic limitations during application, particularly at the site of wastewater generation or in permanent operations. The applications of different AOPs in treating wastewater has been given in Table 5.2. AOPs are required for large critical treatment units to deal with the high COD level to meet strict treatment limits. AOPs have been found to be extremely useful in converting recalcitrant compounds into intermediate compounds that are acquiescent to the biological oxidation process. Among several treatment methods of AOPs, Fenton's reagent has been found to be the most efficient for the treatment of industrial wastewaters containing pollutants like dyes, pesticides, surfactants, organic compounds, etc. One of the advantages of Fenton's reagent is that there is no need for energy to activate hydrogen radicals. Other oxidation processes existing are as follows:

**TABLE 5.2**   Application of Advanced Oxidation Processes (AOPs) in
wastewater treatment

| Methods | Applications | Consequential effects |
|---------|--------------|-----------------------|
| $O_3$ | Removal of Fe and Mn | Increases with increase in ratio of $O_3$ |
| | Control of taste and odor | Efficiently reduces the odd taste and odor |
| | Removing color | Reduction of 70% color from effluents of pulp and paper |
| | Removal of Algae | Helps in removing algae by enhanced filtration method |
| | Helps in disinfection | Process takes place by following removal criteria as bacteria > virus > *Giardia* > *Cryptosporidium* |
| $O_3$-$H_2O_2$ | Control of odor and taste, disinfection, and DBP | Helps in removing ~90% of 2-methylisoborneol and geosmin, reduces DBP formation at the lowest |
| $O_3$-UV | Destruction of micropollutants | Helps in oxidation of trihalomethanes, chloroform, PCBs, bromodichloromethane, Trichloroethylene, etc. |
| $H_2O_2$-UV | Oxidation of SOC | Helps in removing 99% of atrazine from oxidation with its faster rates |

# 5.3.1 The Oxidative Process with Hydrogen Peroxide

This treatment process is an alternative of two systems (i.e., homogeneous and heterogeneous systems). In homogeneous systems, visible light or UV light, soluble catalysts (i.e., Fenton reagents), and ozone or peroxidase-like chemical activators are used; however, clays, semiconductors, zeolites with or without ultraviolet lights are used in heterogeneous systems. Usually, hydrogen peroxides are used as soluble catalysts and are activated by iron salts to form hydroxyl radicals, which are more potent oxidants compared to hydrogen peroxide and ozone. When there is little discharge of wastewater or non-availability of any bio-treatment process at industrial sites, chemical oxidation treatment processes can be recommended instead of installing any central biological effluent treatment plant (Crittenden et al., 1999). The benefits of using these processes are the reduction of effluent color, COD, toxicity, and assistance in removing soluble and insoluble organic substances.

## 5.3.2 The Oxidative Process with Sodium Hypochlorite

In this type of treatment process, the molecules with amino groups are being attacked by the $Cl_2$ and initiates and accelerates the cleavage of azo bonds. During the treatment of dye-containing wastewaters released from textile industries, the increase in the concentration of chlorine molecules favors the decolorization process by removing the dye molecules and decreasing the pH of the wastewater. However, due to the release of aromatic amines and other toxic molecules, this treatment process has found to be inappropriate in removing disperse dyes, eventually becoming less frequent (Mani et al., 2019).

## 5.3.3 Ozonation Process

During this process, ozone—a powerful oxidizing agent—is used to decompose and cleave the aromatic rings of organic pollutants and textile dyes released with industrial wastewaters. The organic pollutants with conjugated double bonds that form smaller molecules with increased toxic and carcinogenic properties are decomposed by ozone and prevents this process. Aside from this, the ozonation process can be used together with physical methods such as adsorption, irradiation, membrane separation, etc. Ozone reacts efficiently—at very low pH through direct reaction pathways—to the chromophoric bonds of molecules, since ozone can be applied at a gaseous state without increasing the volume of sludge or wastewater, proving this process to be beneficial. However, its half-life of ~20 min, destabilization due to the presence of salts, pH, temperature, and installation costs for ozonation plants are considerable disadvantages of this process. Further, the performance of the ozonation process can be improved in combination with membrane filtration technique or irradiation technique.

## 5.3.4 The Photochemical and Electrochemical Oxidation Process

During UV treatments, the presence of $H^+$ decomposes high molecular organic molecules into low weight organic molecules or COO, other inorganic oxides, hydrides, etc. Also, other additional byproducts such as metals, inorganic and organic acids, halides, and organic aldehydes can be produced during treatment based on the original materials and treatment process (Yang et al., 2006). The decomposition of the compounds begins by the formation of hydroxyl and hydroperoxide radicals. The treatment of the wastewater takes place in a batch culture column set-up or in a continuous culture column, where the treatment intensity is influenced by the pH, UV radiation, structure of the compound, and composition. In the photo-oxidation treatment process, the high-performance rate has been reported in the presence of hydrogen peroxide (Anjaneyulu et al., 2005; Zaharia et al., 2009).

The electrochemical oxidation process is considered as an advanced treatment process that offers high removal efficiency for dye-containing industrial wastewaters, especially metal complex dyes, acid dyes, and disperse dyes. Because of its easy set-up, operation, easy control, no additional chemical requirement, and low-temperature work, this procedure has a high-value advantage. The reactors used in this treatment process are highly compact, which prevents the generation of undesirable byproducts. Hypochlorite ion or hypochlorous acid is the primary oxidizing agent used in this process, and these are formed from resulting chloride ions. Other than this, hydroxyl radical and some other reactive species also work as electrochemical oxidation agent directly or indirectly at the anode. This treatment method is considered as an economically efficient approach in treating recycled textile wastewater generated during the dyeing stage. Like other treatment methods, the advantage of this treatment approach is the reduction in the generation of gases, solid wastes, and liquid effluents, but the release of metallic hydroxide sludge is a disadvantage to this method.

## 5.3.5 Comparison between Different Advanced Oxidation Processes

The oxidation of organic compounds is facilitated during the generation of hydroxyl radicals in most advanced oxidation processes (AOPs) helping in the treatment of wastewater by detoxifying the intractable organic and inorganic compounds. Based on several laboratory tests and limited applications in industries, it is assumed that advanced oxidation processes suggest several advantages over existing conventional treatment procedures due to the following reasons:

 i. Are very operational in the process of removing organic compounds;
 ii. If desired, they can completely mineralize the organic contaminants in carbon dioxide;
 iii. They can be resistant to toxic chemicals; and
 iv. Most importantly, less generation of toxic by-products.

Since hydroxyl radicals are not stable in water, the use of AOPs can lower the effect of disinfectant concentration and consequently offer less convenience in microbial sterilization. However, very few pieces of evidence are available on whether complete mineralization of organic compounds is practical on an economic or essential basis. AOPs can also be applied in the pre-treatment process for partial oxidation processes of organic materials—which are either too harmful or resistant to biological degradation. Despite having similarities, each AOP requires a different type of initiators for hydroxyl radical generation, with variation in their generation costs.

Among all the AOPs discussed here, the $O_3$-$H_2O_2$ process is the most comprehensive application due to its low cost and high efficacy. The $H_2O_2$-UV process is very simple, since only $H_2O_2$ chemical is required for this process, can easily be stored for a long time, costs only 30% of the solution, and can be used in the process only at a demand of the metering pump, which gives this process a distinctive advantage. $H_2O_2$ is a miscible liquid that gets mixed with water without creating any problem during transfers, making this process advantageous for small systems requiring minimal maintenance, discontinuous operation, or both. Sometimes, the materials in water may intensely absorb UV rays making the $H_2O_2$-UV process less effective because of the lagging of radical reaction instigation (Zhou and Smith, 2002).

At higher pH, the consumption of ozone has restricted usage as it requires a large quantity of neutralizing chemicals—that's why the $O_3$-UV process is less preferred than the $O_3$-$H_2O_2$ and $H_2O_2$-UV processes. However, when the pollutants have strong UV absorbance capacity to be oxidized, then these ozonation based processes can be applied at low flow rates. Lastly, the least used processes are a photo-catalytic process that also offers various advantages like no additional $H_2O_2$ requirement, reusable photocatalysts, and use of natural radiations as a source of light for activating catalysts. Currently, these processes undergo low quantum production for radical initiation.

# 5.4 BIOAUGMENTATION

The toxic organic pollutants in industrial effluents or activated sludge are biologically degraded using microorganisms. However, there are few overly complex structured pollutants that do not easily get degenerated and are resistant to biodegradability in wastewater. To overcome these restrictions, bioaugmentation strategies or processes are used. Bioaugmentation is a process that has the capacity to biodegrade recalcitrant pollutants, along with microorganisms, which contaminate our environment (Semrany et al., 2012). When compared with physico-chemical treatment approaches, the bioaugmentation process is found to be cost-effective as well as eco-friendly (Figure 5.1). Different bioaugmentation approaches have been reviewed, including challenges that occur during wastewater treatments (Herrero and Stuckey, 2015).

Despite unpredictable bioaugmentation outcomes, it has been emphasized in agricultural and wastewater treatment plants for years. When compared with other wastewater treatment processes, this process is still thought to be less predictable and better regulated as it results in the demolition of toxic pollutants (Boon et al., 2000). The bioaugmentation

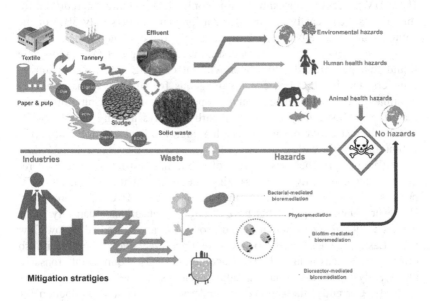

**FIGURE 5.1**   Different types of pollutants source and mitigation strategies.

process takes advantage of using different microbial consortia, which were designed for specific physico-chemical possessions of bioprocess, because this approach was found to be more efficient than utilizing undecided inocula.

## 5.4.1 Removal of Recalcitrant Pollutants from Industrial Wastewater

Industrial wastewaters consist of naturally occurring microorganisms that have the capacity of degrading a range of pollutants; however, pollutants that are non-biodegradable are also present in the effluent. Low water solubility, low bioavailability, high stability, high toxicity, and low biodegradability—along with some compounds that are not utilized efficiently in the form of substrates by metabolic enzyme activity of microbes—are some factors that make pollutants resistant (Chandra and Chowdhary, 2015). Certain pollutants comprised of complex chemical structures require different microorganisms for its degradation, but at the same time, it's not necessary that all microorganisms are present in the environment. Sometimes, new recalcitrant compounds get generated into the wastewater, and microorganisms have yet to adapt to those compounds as their substrate (Providenti et al., 1993). The bioaugmentation process is used to overcome these challenges as one of the advantages of this treatment technology is that it can be personalized according to the dominant pollutant in the environment. Thus, this treatment technology is regarded as an appealing approach when dealing with both pollutants in higher concentrations and emerging pollutants in increasing numbers. Several researchers have been focused on testing the bioaugmentation treatment technology strategies in the cleaning of wastewaters by keeping an eye on recalcitrant pollutants from over the last decade.

## 5.4.2 Applications of Bioaugmentation In Removing Different Pollutants

### 5.4.2.1 Removal of Chlorinated and Fluorinated Compounds

Halogenated compounds have been utilized in several ways such as adhesives, degreasing agents, fungicides, lubricants, plastic components, pesticides, and wood preservatives (Mattes et al., 2010). In a study in

2012, it was estimated that a total of 764,000 $m^3$ tons of chlorinated solvents were used worldwide both in industries and at homes, leading to wastewater contamination—which bioaugmentation treatment methods have efficiently removed (Loffler et al., 2013). In an experiment with synthetic wastewater medium supplemented with activated sludge (AS), it was shown that the bacteria *Acinetobacter* sp. TW and *Comamonas testosterone* I2 were found to biodegrade 4-fluoroaniline and 3-chloroaniline, respectively, with optimum conditions favoring colonization and biofilm formation that increased the significant rate of biodegradation (Boon et al., 2000; Wang et al., 2013). In another study in a laboratory, 2,4-dichlorophenol was biodegraded by bioaugmentation method with the bacterial consortium in synthetic wastewater medium enriched with activated sludge (Quan et al., 2004). Puyol et al. (2015) reported increased biodegradation of 2,4,6-trichlorophenol after bioaugmentation with *Desulfito bacterium* sp. by using a fluidized bed biofilm reactor (FBBR) and expanded granular sludge bed (EGSB). These studies were made only in laboratory settings; therefore, the removal of these halogenated compounds at full-scale wastewater treatment plants by bioaugmentation still a matter of concern.

### 5.4.2.2 Removal of Lignin Compound

Another experiment successfully conducted is the degrading of lignin compounds from the paper industry through bioaugmentation. Pulp and paper industries generate a huge volume of wastewaters known as black liquor, which has high lignin content. It is estimated that for a production of one ton of pulp, around seven tons of wastewater is generated (Biermann, 1993; Zainith et al., 2019). Along with lignin, black liquor consists of polysaccharides and resinous compounds. Since lignin-degrading microorganisms are not commonly found in pulp and paper wastewater, natural biological treatment with activated sludge is not efficient in removing all these compounds (Wu et al., 2005). To remove specific pollutants originating in black liquor, the selection and addition of potent lignin-biodegrading microorganisms into wastewaters is a sensible strategy (Chowdhary et al., 2020b; Zainith et al., 2020). A microbial consortium consisting of *Comamonas* B-9 and *Pandoraea* B-6 (bacteria) and *Aspergillus* F-1 (Fungus) was prepared by isolating from AS through sequence batch reactor (SBR) and was tested in degrading lignocellulose compounds. Their results suggested that at a laboratory scale, bioaugmented AS enhanced the lignin removal ~>50%, consisting of SBR with a working volume of 2 L (Zhang et al., 2013). This research showed that bioaugmentation could be an alternative process in enhancing the biological treatment of lignin-containing wastewater.

### 5.4.2.3 Removal of Cyanides

One of the most toxic compounds released from the steel industry by burning coal during the cooking process is cyanides; therefore, it is necessary to treat the industrial wastewater before their disposal. The biological removal of cyanides can be enhanced by adding cyanide-degrading yeast *Cryptococcus humicolus* and an unidentified microorganism constituting ferric cyanide into wastewater through the bioaugmentation process. However, this process proved to be less efficient in biodegrading ferric cyanide in wastewater because of the poor settling process and slow biodegradation. Therefore, more study is needed on this approach to make it more efficient in removing cyanides from wastewater (Park et al., 2008).

### 5.4.2.4 Removal of Diethylene Glycol Monobutyl Ether

Polar solvents such as glycol ethers, glycol monobutyl ether, and diethylene glycol monobutyl ether (DGBE) can easily mix with water and organic chemicals and are most used in cleaners and paints. These solvents have shown toxic effects on animal models, are very cumbersome during biodegradation, and strongly accumulate in the environment after being discharged in industrial wastewaters. Chen et al. (2016) studied the potentiality of *Serratia* sp. strain isolated from contaminated wastewater of the silicon plate industry on the removal of DGBE with bioaugmentation and found an increased rate of DGBE removal rate both at the laboratory and full-scale level (Sitarek et al., 2012).

### 5.4.2.5 Removal of Nicotine

Nicotine, a carcinogen, is released in the wastewaters from tobacco industries along with other toxic substances. For a ton of cigarettes, 60 tons of contaminated wastewaters are released into the environment (Zhong et al., 2010). The bioaugmentation process is evaluated as a strong strategy for removing these pollutants and several microorganisms (*Acinetobacter* sp. and *Sphingomonas* sp.) that have been identified as capable of biodegrading nicotine (Wang et al., 2011). Wang et al. (2013) studied the bioaugmentation effect with *Acinetobacter* sp. on nicotine biodegradation and found increased nicotine removal from ~10% in a controlled reactor to 98% in a bioaugmented reactor. Comparable results were also reported with another nicotine biodegrading bacterial strain *Pseudomonas* sp. HF-1 is a sequence batch reactor showing bioaugmentation benefits in nicotine removal (Wang et al., 2009). However, these studies were made on a small scale, and to date, no report is available showing a study on tobacco wastewater treatment plants.

## 5.4.2.6 Removal of Polycyclic Aromatic Hydrocarbons and Heterocyclic Compounds

Polycyclic Aromatic hydrocarbons (PAHs) are another type of pollutants found frequently in industrial wastewaters—in petroleum products, coal conversion industries, and organic material synthesis. Polycyclic aromatic compounds are recalcitrant compounds that do not degrade and persists in the environment for an extended period, consequently causing toxic and hazardous effects on humans and the environment. One of the most toxic PAHs is a naphthalene compound. Its removal test was performed using *Streptomyces* sp. strain through bioaugmentation in the wastewater of coal gasification in a membrane bioreactor, and results showed its significant elimination from wastewater (Xu et al., 2015). Zhu et al. (2015) performed a similar test on the bioaugmentation of cooking wastewater with a developed consortium of five strains of *Pseudomonas* sp. and *Paracoccus denitificans* and this bioaugmentation process assisted the removal of pollutants carbazole, naphthalene, phenol, pyridine, and quinoline found in cooking wastewater. In another study, phenol present in wastewater from coal gasification was removed using a mixture of phenol-degrading bacterial on biological contact oxidation reactor, but the bacterial species name was not revealed (Fang et al., 2013).

## 5.4.2.7 Removal of Pyridine and Quinoline Compounds

Pyridines and quinolines are *N*-heterocyclic compounds that are used as solvents for paints, dyes, and wood treating chemicals and are found as raw materials in pharmaceutical and industrial wastes and, subsequently, in industrial wastewaters. Quinolines—carcinogenic compounds—are recalcitrant compounds that are commonly found in coal tar and petroleum products. They persist in the environment because of their low biodegradability. In a study, enhanced biodegradation of quinoline present in petroleum refinery wastewater was reported by using *Bacillus* sp., which was isolated from the soil through the batch reactor (Tuo et al., 2012). In another study, pyridine and quinoline were successfully biodegraded by *Paracoccus* sp. and *Pseudomonas* sp. bioaugmented with wastewater medium. In this study, though, the level of pyridine and quinoline was reduced, but the nitrogen content was reported to remain high (Bai et al., 2009). To overcome this challenge, another study was performed using the same microorganisms in an SBR reactor with modified zeolite, which contributed to the removal of nitrogen through adsorption and results showed reduced pyridine, quinoline, and nitrogen content in the medium (Bai et al., 2010). The increased removal of pyridine was also reported through the bioaugmentation of industrial wastewater using SBR with *Rhizobium* sp. and in a membrane batch reactor (MBR) with *Paracoccus denitrificans* (Liu et al., 2015; Wen et al., 2013). To date, no further study has been reported in the removal of pyridine and quinoline.

### 5.4.2.8 Removal of Synthetic Dyes

Primarily used synthetic dyes are azo and anthraquinone based molecules that are used on a wide range in textile industries, and ~7 × 10$^5$ tons of dyes are produced yearly. Among these dyes, it is estimated that ~2–10% can contaminate the environment through industrial wastewater (Fan et al., 2008). One of the largest and diverse groups of dyes is azo dyes, which are found to be resistant to biodegradation with conventional activated sludge treatment methods (Pandey et al., 2007). Increased removal of an azo dye, Acid Orange 7, was reported through bioaugmentation with *Shewanella* sp. XB in a membrane aerated biofilm reactor (Wang et al., 2012). To produce anthraquinone dyes, bromoamine acid (BAA)—a very toxic and recalcitrant compound—is required as a major intermediate product. To produce dye, industries produce BAA, which contaminates wastewaters. Therefore, BAA biodegrading strain *Sphingomonas* sp. was isolated and bioaugmented with micro-electrolysis and biological aerated filtration process of wastewater (Fan et al., 2008, 2009). Still, a successful study is needed for the removal of synthetic dyes at the full scale of treatment plants.

## 5.4.3 Limitations of Bioaugmentation Process Treatment

The treatment of industrial wastewaters through bioaugmentation has been extensively and successfully used at a laboratory scale with very encouraging outcomes, but these results have not yet been applied on full-scale wastewater treatment plants. Along with the successful removal of pollutants from both soil and water (surface and ground) by the bioaugmentation process, a number of failures of the bioaugmentation process have also been reported (Kalogerakis, 2016; Stroo et al., 2013). When studying full-scale wastewater treatment plants, researchers observed a decrease in the number of exogenous microorganisms as soon they are added to any site. Several factors have been explained as a reason for the death of microorganisms—which includes biotic and abiotic stresses. These stressors occur due to competition between introduced and indigenous microorganisms, temperature changes, pH, insufficient substrates, nutrient limitations, phase infections, grazing by protozoa, pollutant load shock, and quorum sensing (QS), which might be a reason to full-scale wastewater treatment failures. Apart from all these, one successful full-scale bioaugmentation treatment method has been reported for in-situ removal of chlorinated solvents—mainly chlorinated ethenes—from groundwater by using the Dehalococcoides group of anaerobic bacteria (Bouchez et al., 2000; Stroo et al., 2013). To overcome these limitations, documented evidence on failures and strategies of bioaugmentation can be used in the future.

# 5.5 ALGAL TREATMENT

The amount of wastewaters increased along with population growth accompanied by greater water utilization due to urbanization and industrialization. This is the top reason for the rapid increase in water pollution and one of the critical environmental problems to be focused on. In most developing countries like India, the conventional methods for the treatment of industrial wastewaters are too costly non-economical therefor, so green technological methods are being opted and introduced to solve the issues related with conventional technologies (Bharagava and Chowdhary, 2018; Chowdhary et al., 2020a) An example of a green technology that has gained importance is the application of microalgae. It has been accepted worldwide for the last 50 years and is found to be as effective as other conventional treatment methods (Sen et al., 2013). Nowadays, microalgae are used as a potential biological agent for the treatment of industrial wastewater as well as an alternative source of energy. This treatment is one of the best and most trusted technologies in treating environmental-related problems such as climate change—by consuming high $CO_2$ levels produced during photosynthesis and producing oxygen and glucose—global warming, and the increased ozone hole (Ahmad et al., 2012). It can utilize different sources such as carbon dioxide, sunlight, and various other nutrients in removing organic and inorganic toxic compounds, heavy metals, nutrients, and other impurities present in industrial wastewater.

One of the advantage of algal treatment system is that they absorb harmful solar radiation and use them as a source of energy in their chloroplast cells; they utilize carbon dioxide along with other nutrients present in wastewater to synthesize their biomass and produce oxygen. To metabolize the residual organic compounds, present in the treated industrial wastewater through aerobic bacterial systems, the oxygen produced by these microalgae is found to be more sufficient. Algae release simple organic materials in massive amounts, which can be adapted for the aqueous system. At the same time, bacteria consist of carbon dioxide, which promotes algal growth and encourages the release of organic growth factors and vitamins and maintains pH level for the growth of algae (Sekaran et al., 2013). The relation between the maximum yields of biomass regarding biological nutrients (which can be consumed either wholly or partially depending on the nutritional value present in a water body) used for algal growth is determined through Algal Growth Potential (AGP) (Travieso et al., 1999). The effluents are rich in nutrients that are generated from any industry, which should be treated well before discharge into any water body where they can cause eutrophication. However, this recycling process increases the overall cost and might disrupt the full treatment process due to the accumulation of phosphorus. To overcome this situation, a possible solution is the incorporation or growth of algae (since it grows very well in wastewater and can treat nutrient-rich wastewater) by utilizing carbon dioxide gas released from the chimney of power plant (Omatoyo et al., 2013). This capability of the algal system to grow in nutrient-rich wastewater (nitrogen, phosphorus, and other minerals) can help treat various types of wastewaters—domestic, agricultural, sewage, municipal, and other industrial wastewaters—generated vigorously. This microalgae-based treatment method shows several benefits since these are aquatic microorganisms that do not require any type of cultivational land for their growth. Indeed, microalgae can be cultivated with fewer uses in a minimal land, and water used during cultivation can be fresh, saline, or even waste—twice the seawater concentration of salt can be used very effectively (Matthew, 2008).

## 5.5.1 Factors Affecting Microalgae Growth

### 5.5.1.1 Sunlight

Since microalgae are unicellular photosynthetic microorganisms, it requires sunlight energy for growth. They utilize sunlight and convert it into organic molecules (carbohydrates). The absence of sunlight reduces the growth of microalgae.

### 5.5.1.2 Carbon Dioxide ($CO_2$)

Carbon Dioxide is a significant contributor to global warming because of its daily increase in atmospheric level, but its potential effects are still being understood (Yafei, 2014). Microalgae use sunlight and carbon dioxide to prepare their food through photosynthetic activity, and in return, release oxygen into the environment. Microalgae not only utilizes atmospheric carbon dioxide but also fixes $CO_2$ from different other sources such as industrial released gases, wastewaters, and soluble carbonates as their source of carbon for growth. According to Yafei (2014), ~50% of carbon is contained in the microalgal cells from which 1 kg of biomass is produced by fixing 1.8 kg of carbon dioxide—which is why they are considered to be more efficient than terrestrial plants in fixing $CO_2$.

### 5.5.1.3 Nutrient Sources

The utilization of nutrient-rich industrial and municipal wastewaters as a source of feedstock in the production of microalga has met with economical and eco-friendly benefits (Belinda and Stacey, 2011). Microalgae are fed into the wastewater consisting of nutrients like phosphorus, sulfur, nitrogen, iron, toxins, and heavy metals to produce microbial biomass. Among these nutrients, nitrogen and phosphorus (after $CO_2$) are considered to be the most vital for microalgae growth. Microalgae use phosphorus as a source of inorganic compound (in the form of orthophosphate) for their growth (Karin, 2006). Wastewater consists of all types of macronutrients and micronutrients, helping the growth of microalgae.

### 5.5.1.4 pH

The pH level of wastewater may affect the growth of microalgae and the treatment process of wastewaters. The pH level regulates the availability of specific types of inorganic carbon sources, and if the pH level increases for any reason, then photosynthetic carbon dioxide gets exhausted (Karin, 2006). Also, high pH and dissolved oxygen concentration cause phosphorus sedimentation and removal of hydrogen sulfur as well as ammonia, whereas in algal ponds, high pH leads to pathogen disinfection. Studies on cyanobacterium *Anabaena variabilis* reported that at pH 8.2–8.4, the optimal productivity is obtained, while a pH of 7.4–7.8, slightly lower, and decreased growth has been reported at pH above 9. The cells of cyanobacterium were found to be unable to grow at pH 9.7–9.9 (Fontes et al., 1987).

### 5.5.1.5 Temperature

Temperature plays an important role during microalgal growth because an increase in temperature might increase the photosynthesis rate, which enhances the algal biomass. Too much light might lower the photosynthetic effectivity, which is known as photoinhibition. Algal growth increases with temperature, until the optimum level is obtained. Further increase might lead to rapid growth reduction of algae. For maximum algal growth, the optimized temperature is reported to be between 20 and 30 °C.

## 5.6 MISCELLANEOUS METHODS

Among other biological treatment approaches described below, there are few green technologies applied for the remediation of industrial wastewaters containing a variety of pollutants.

### 5.6.1 Engineered Wetlands

These are the manmade wetland systems that are eco-friendly and were planned for removing highly recalcitrant toxic products from the wastewaters generated from different industries into the environment. These wetlands are constructed by utilizing the naturally occurring bio-geochemical processing of the soil microbes and treating the industrial wastewaters with them to recover the wastewater with useful nutrient qualities. Plant-associated microorganisms play an essential role in the constructed wetlands, which helps in the degradation and detoxification of the recalcitrant toxic pollutants into less toxic compounds (Kabra et al., 2012). This process is the most appealing and profitable approach in the remediation of a wide range of waste products discharged along with different types of industrial wastewaters. The wetlands are rich in rhizospheric microorganisms, which play a significant role in removing non-essential nutrients and contaminants like heavy metals from the industrial wastewater being used for treatment (Bai et al., 2014). Along with microorganisms, some aquatic macrophytes such as *Azolla, Eichornia, Typha,* etc., are found to be capable in removing or detoxifying heavy metal contaminants in wetlands.

### 5.6.2 Bioremediation

The bioremediation process is the most effective, eco-friendly, and cost-effective approach for the management of harmful and toxic pollutants containing industrial wastewaters. This process utilizes metabolic potentials of naturally occurring living agents—principally microorganisms—for degrading and reducing toxic pollutants into less toxic products through mineralization under in-situ or ex-situ conditions. Bioremediation is a terminology describing various environmental-friendly techniques such as composting, bio-stimulation, rhizofiltration, bioaugmentation, bioventing, bioleaching, land-farming, etc. To get the benefits from the bioremediation process, microorganisms must grow and survive in a polluted atmosphere where are affected by a variety of biotic and abiotic factors directly or indirectly. The bioremediation process takes place in three phases: in the first phase, toxic industrial wastes are reduced by naturally occurring indigenous microorganisms such as *Bacillus, Pseudomonas, Micrococcus, Mycobacterium*, etc. In the second phase, nutrients and oxygen are supplied to enhance the efficacy of the biodegradation process; while in the third phase, other microbes are added to the system to further increase the efficacy and degradation of the targeted toxicants (Megharaj et al., 2011).

## 5.6.3 Phytoremediation

For the removal and degradation of industrial wastewater pollutants, an alternative technology known as phytoremediation or plant-mediated remediation is being used, which utilizes the whole plant or their specific parts for treatment. This whole technology is a plant-based green technology that can accumulate substantial concentrations of poisonous chemicals. Phytoremediation technology involves five different physiological plant mechanisms—phytoextraction, rhizofiltration, phytostabilization, phytodegradation, and phytovolatilization. It is an innovative technology that helps in understanding the plant-microbe association and uses mutualism in establishing a healthy relationship in the rhizospheric region of plants for detoxification or degradation of lethal pollutants from the environment. Plants such as *Arbidopsis* sp., *Sedum alfredii* sp., and *Thlapsi* sp. has been reported to be hyperaccumulators, which have great potential in accumulating high concentrations of harmful metals and translocating them into parts of plants that can easily be harvested for maximum reduction of pollutants (Kabeer et al., 2014). The use of these plants is proven to be a cost-effective and abundantly available method, which has provided substantial assistance in creating a pollution-free and green environment (Figure 5.1).

# Merits and Demerits of Conventional vs. New Technologies

# 6

Water pollution is defined as pollution created in water by adding one or more constituents that modify water in a way that causes problems to humans, animals, and the environment. The major concern of water pollution is the chemicals with it, which has become a priority for society and public specialists and, most importantly, the industrial world responsible for these problems. The prime cause of water pollution is the release of chemicals with other toxic materials from multiple sources (chemical fertilizers, energy use, industrial wastes, pesticides, mining activities, radioactive wastes, sewage and wastes, urban development, etc.). The fact is that water is used at every step of each process—whether agricultural, domestic, or industrial—which produces contaminated water. Therefore, a constant effort should be made to protect water resources.

In developing countries, the legislation is becoming extremely strict regarding the release of industrial wastewater and has imposed treatment processes before their disposal into the environment. Recently, in Europe, guidelines have been established for the protection of surface water, underground water, and coastal water. Industrial sectors should innovate and reduce or eliminate the dangerous and priority substances from the wastewater before their release. In the context of sustainable development, the recycling of effluents is gaining active attention from industries as better waste management towards health concerns. Simple wastewater treatment technologies can be designed to provide low-cost sanitation and environmental protection while providing additional benefits from the reuse of water. Therefore, the treatment of effluent should be a top priority. Several conventional and modern technologies—including physical, chemical, and biological processes—have been reported during the past three decades, such as floatation, oxidation, adsorption, membrane filtration, biodegradation, bioaugmentation, etc. All these processes have their own merits and demerits, not only in cost but also in efficiency, viability, and environmental impact. Presently, no single process is considered as an adequate treatment because of the complex nature of the effluents released. However, the combination of one or more methods usually achieve desirable water quality in an economical way.

# 6.1 AVAILABLE TECHNOLOGIES FOR REMOVING POLLUTANTS

Established conventional wastewater treatment processes to remove solid pollutants are combinations of physical, chemical, and biological processes that help reduce or eliminate soluble contaminants, nutrients, organic and inorganic materials, etc. from effluents. Apart from these technologies, new emerging methods—including reverse osmosis, membrane filtration, bioaugmentation, algal treatments, etc.—has been established to obtain a higher quality of liquid effluent, which can be recycled. The selection of any conventional or modern treatment method depends on the characteristics of the effluent discharged and, most importantly, less consumption.

In the current scenario, the development of a cheaper, effective, and innovative method for the treatment of industrial wastewater/effluent is an active research area of interest according to the numerous publications during recent years. At present, protecting the environment—particularly problems related to water pollution—has become the primary concern of the public, industrialists, scientists, researchers, and decision-makers at national and international levels. Due to the public demand on pollutant-free effluents discharged from industries to the receiving water bodies, their treatment and decontamination has now become top priorities—which is a complicated and challenging task. The development of any universal and new method used to examine and eliminate all contaminants/pollutants from wastewaters is even more difficult. This book describes the merits as well as demerits of all technologies (such as conventional and recent emerging methods) available for the wastewater treatment processes, as described in Table 6.1.

**TABLE 6.1** Merits and demerits of conventional and emerging wastewater treatment technologies

| Technology Conventional methods | Characteristics | Merits | Demerits |
|---|---|---|---|
| Chemical precipitation | Pollutant uptake and separation of products formed | Simple, Integrated physiochemical process, Economical and efficient, Adopted to high pollutant loads, Efficient for metal and fluoride elimination, Significant reduction in chemical oxygen demand | Consumption of chemicals like $H_2S$, lime, etc., Effluents physico-chemical analysis, Low concentration removal of metal ions is ineffective and oxidation process is required in case of complex metals Production of high sludge resulting in management and disposal problems |
| Sedimentation | Separation of products | Helps in efficient destruction of non-biodegradable effluents as well as toxic wastes | Efficient in removing only large microorganisms and settleable solids such as silts, sands, etc. |
| Coagulation/ flocculation | Pollutant uptake and separation of products formed | Simple process assimilated with physico-chemical methods including a wide range of low-cost chemicals which are easily available, Lessens inefficient removal of suspended solids and colloidal particles as well as reduces BOD and COD, Efficiently reduces TOC, insoluble contaminants, and AOX from the pulp and paper industry | Joining of non-reusable chemicals are required, Effluents physico-chemical analysis is required Generation of sludge in large volume increases and removal of arsenic becomes low |

*(Continued)*

TABLE 6.1 (Continued)

| Technology | Characteristics | Merits | Demerits |
|---|---|---|---|
| **Conventional methods** | | | |
| Trickling filters | Removal of organic materials | Low requirement of land and can be used as a small-scale treatment | Machine-driven equipment are required |
| Activated sludge | Helps in the removal of heavy metals and pollution loads | Low requirement of land and are a highly efficient technique for treatment | Costly procedure and requires a large area for disposal of sludge |
| Rotating biological contactors | Removal of nitrogen and biodegradable organic materials | Are the most efficient treatment technique and can be operated in a small land, Can be applied as both small- and large-scale treatment method | Not cost-effective and demands highly trained staff for maintenance and operation of devices, Also require high energy and spare parts |
| **Emerging Technologies** | | | |
| Reverse osmosis | Separation is non-destructive through semi-permeable barriers | Availability of membranes from numerous manufacturers, Requires little space, Rapid and efficient at high concentrations with generation of less solid wastes | Requires high energy and capital for maintenance and operation |
| Membrane filtration | Separation of differently sized molecules | Helpful in recycling of water | Filtration membrane fouls and are found to be inefficient in reducing solid contents |

TABLE 6.1 (Continued)

| Technology Conventional methods | Characteristics | Merits | Demerits |
|---|---|---|---|
| Oxidation process | An emerging but destructive technique | Produces reactive radicals in-situ by consuming little amount of chemicals, Causes mineralization of pollutants without sludge production, Recalcitrant compounds are rapidly degraded | Found to be financially impractical in small and medium industry, Produces by-products at industrial scale |
| Algal treatment | Stops eutrophication by utilizing phosphorus and nitrogen for their growth | Helps in decreasing the ration of pollutants and pathogen, Nutrients are recovered in the form of valuable biomass, Saves energy and less emission of $CO_2$ | Requires large land, The physico-chemical characteristics of the effluent affects its activity, Environmental conditions influence, Harvesting of biomass and volarization |
| Bioaugmentation | Enhances the microbial populations of the contaminated site | Are cost-effective and requires less labor, Causes less harmful impact on the environment, Helps treat the contaminated soils and groundwater with chlorinated solvents | Microbes need an ideal environment to thrive the process efficiently, Requires an extended period, Bacteria cannot metabolize all types of wastes |

(Continued)

TABLE 6.1 (Continued)

| Technology Conventional methods | Characteristics | Merits | Demerits |
|---|---|---|---|
| **Miscellaneous Methods** | | | |
| Engineered wetlands | Removal of a wide range of bacterial contaminants | Up to 70% removal of solids and bacteria, Requires less capital, Maintenance and handling cost are minimal | Requires management of extra plant materials and suitable for places where native plants are easily available |
| Bioremediation | Uses microbes to degrade contaminants | Efficient in converting and reducing highly toxic and hazardous compounds into less toxic compounds | Have application limitations to only biodegradable compounds |
| Phytoremediation | Utilizes green living plants to clean contaminated soil and groundwater | More cost-effective than other traditional processes both in-situ and ex-situ, Valuable metals can be recovered and reused, Use of plants reduces soil erosion and leaching of metals | Not effective in sites with higher concentration of contaminants, Slower than other conventional techniques, Season variation affects its process |

# Prospects of New Technologies

7

In emerging and developing countries, a shortage of technical staff for handling operations and maintenance is one of the critical challenges the increasing water demand. In this process, several emerging industrial wastewater treatment technologies have been reviewed on both laboratory scale and practical applications to demonstrate that these methods have a broad-spectrum capacity of reducing biological as well as chemical contaminants, which were very difficult to remove through existing conventional wastewater treatment technologies. Some of these processes are found to be advance in equipment manufacturing and their regulatory requirements and are of incredibly competitive pricing. To remove organic and inorganic compounds and separate solid-liquid combination, membrane filtration processes are highly effective. In the near future—even if desalination by RO will remain an essential application in the treatment of wastewater or water—treatments like microfiltration (MF) and ultrafiltration (UF) will be utilized for the disinfection of resistant microorganisms such as *Cryptosporidium* sp. and *Giardia* sp. during the removal of disinfection by-products.

A better understanding regarding the key issues in membrane processes—better membrane materials and module designs, membrane integrity mechanism, membrane fouling mechanisms, and more effective fouling control strategies—should be improved for advancement. To remove chlorine-resistant microbial contaminants, an alternative disinfectant technology—ozone—has been widely used to reduce color, control odor and taste, oxidize synthetic organic compounds, and destabilize particles during wastewater treatment. Several new advanced oxidation processes (AOPs) have been developed by combining ozone treatment technology with hydrogen peroxide, UV, sodium hypochlorite, and heterogeneous photocatalysts. Still, most of these processes are for improvement since these are remarkably effective in the oxidation of intractable organic pollutants. Further research is required to understand and control by-products such as bromate and bromated organic compounds generated during the ozonation process. AOP efficiency should be improved in carrying out the oxidation of organic contaminants. For the reduction of bacterial indicator organisms in wastewater, the most used treatment is ultraviolet radiation and, according to recent investigations, it has been found particularly useful in eliminating *Cryptosporidium*. If this is true, then the application of UV irradiation will expand rapidly in the treatment of industrial wastewater. A hybrid treatment technology has recently been suggested, which is formed by combining conventional treatment methods with advanced treatment processes, and some samples of these hybrid technologies—AOPs-biodegradation, membrane bioreactor, membrane-PAC—have been included and are under surveillance. If used properly, these hybrid processes might become the most effective and economical approach in the future for dealing with existing environmental problems (Chowdhary et al., 2018c, 2020b) Still, further research regarding synergistic and adverse effects is needed to better understand these hybrid technologies.

At present, the research and technical issues regarding the management of wastewater can be grouped into the following areas.

## 7.1 UPGRADING WASTEWATER TREATMENT PLANTS (WWTPS)

Most wastewater treatment plants were established more than two decades ago; they need to be upgraded to improve their capacity and treatment efficiency. Such revamp might help utilize the emerging technologies or establish one in a better or newer form. Some of the current and future interests are as follows:

- Development of innovative wastewater collection system designs;
- Calculation of long-term performance and lifetime cost-effectiveness of emerging treatment technologies equipped with new as well as existing materials; and
- Development of a treatment system which utilizes less energy and minimizes the emission of greenhouse gases.

# 7.2 RECOVERY OF ENERGY AND NUTRIENTS

The nutrients present in industrial wastewaters are responsible for the excessive algal growth and ammonia production in the receiving water body, causing toxic effects on aquatic life. Therefore, technologies capable of removing nutrients from wastewaters are an essential research objective. New sustainable technology capable of reducing nutrient concentration with minimized cost, energy, and chemical consumption should be introduced. The development of full-scale anaerobic MBRs to meet requirements of secondary and advanced treatment techniques should be optimized for various operating conditions and climates to meet the standards of reclaimed water with disinfection. Optimization and application of nitritation-denitration and deammonification evaluating operations should be improved to promote nitrite-oxidizing bacteria (NOB) and treat low temperatures of mainstream wastewater. New processes should also be developed; understanding the ratio of organic nitrogen in the effluent and minimize its production. Analytical methods should also be improved to measure the deficient levels of phosphorus, and innovative technologies should be developed for the recovery of resources like carbon, water, nutrients from wastewater, and enhanced anaerobic digestion and processes for conversion of other solids.

# 7.3 REMOVAL OF OTHER CONTAMINANTS

Endocrine Disrupting Compounds (EDCs) are compounds that change the endocrine system and causes adverse effect on humans and wildlife. Highly persisting pharmaceutical compounds and their metabolites have been reported as pharmaceutically active compounds (PhACs) and are known to function as EDCs. Therefore, the development of modern technologies is required for cost-effective removal, prevention, and reduction of these EDCs, PhACs, prions, etc. introduced into wastewater. The development of sustainable and improved disinfectant technology is required to control pathogens such as *E. coli-0157, Cryptosporidium, Giardia*, etc., and other microorganisms without disinfecting the by-products generated. The emerging and innovative technologies for the removal of promising pollutants from water and wastewater should be developed with minimal cost and energy.

## 7.4 SECURITY OF WATER SYSTEMS

New wastewater treatment systems must be prepared for emergencies like pandemics, spill incidents, or new bacterial or viral strain. New WWT systems should be capable of improvement strategies after any natural calamity and should also prepare and prevent against bioterrorism.

## 7.5 CONSERVATION OF ENERGY AND RENEWABLE ENERGY SOURCES

New wastewater treatment processes should be more energy efficient in processing and operating techniques. To become self-sufficient in energy, most wastewater facilities are searching for some cost-effective renewable energy sources, which includes hydropower, solar cells, fuel cells, wind turbines, and extraction of heat from industrial wastewaters. The production of digester gas should be increased and must be appropriately utilized to generate heat and electric power onsite. For commercial purposes, clean biogas should be exported.

## 7.6 OPTIMIZATION OF WASTEWATER AND SOLID TREATMENTS

The optimization processes for treating both wastewaters and solids might reduce the costs involved in energy, maintenance, human resources, and other operational techniques. The cost-effective methods should also be developed to minimize the volume and quantity of wastewaters and solids generated during production, without reducing the value or quality of the products. New recovery methods should involve the successful reuse of bio-solids and wastewaters generated during production.

# 7.7 ALTERNATIVE REMEDIATION TECHNOLOGIES

Despite the tremendous advances in conventional and innovative technologies based on bioremediation, environmental concern still exists, and such challenges lead to alternative technologies for effective bioremediation. Predictive or *in silico* bioremediation is an emerging technology for remediation of contaminants when conventional bioremediation fail to perform (Chowdhary et al., 2020a). Different computational techniques are the soul of predictive bioremediation, relying on computational tools and techniques, predicting the possible degradation pathways, binding affinity, and predicting dynamics for quick understanding of enzyme ligand interactions. Such functionalities could transform the existing field of conventional bioremediation (Singh et al., 2020).

# Conclusion

**8**

One of the most critical primary mechanisms of settlement configuration is the supply and safe disposal of industrial wastewaters. Currently, it can be seen clearly that due to the scarcity of freshwater and lack of sanitary facilities, the rate of illness and death is increasing daily. Tons of freshwaters are required by several industries for carrying out production processes—and most of these waters are released into the environment in the form of wastewaters. To meet the daily requirements for water, health, and other resource protection, the demand for viable wastewater treatment technologies need further development and implementations (Schaum et al., 2015a). In an account, there are many questions regarding ecology, economy, technology, and society which have to be taken seriously, and our future development must focus on these topics described below (Schaum and Cornel, 2016):

- *Water Protection:* For the protection of different water sources, the released industrial wastewaters in the environment should be treated before discharge to eliminate nutrients in its greatest extent, to protect receiving water bodies from eutrophication. Along with this, microplastics, micropollutants, and nanoparticles should also be eliminated from the effluents discharged.
- *Health Protection:* To fulfill the daily hygiene requirements, disinfection measures should be taken for water bodies with treated wastewaters before their reuse, and water should also be preserved from antibiotic-resistant microorganisms.
- *Resource Protection:* A multipurpose resource-efficient operation should be launched to utilize resources such as water, energy, and nutrients present in the wastewaters. By minimizing the emission of certain greenhouse gases, climate protection can be initiated.

Based on several case studies reported, a deep discussion should be done on the risk factors and requirements for removal of certain groups of toxic chemical pollutants and their cost-benefit ratios from the industrial wastewaters, which are released into the environment on a daily basis. However, before making any decision on a specific technology that can solve the acute problems, all up-coming requirements should be considered within the scope of vital planning; otherwise, this might hinder the path in response, which may challenge our future needs. The cooperation effects should always be kept in mind. For ex-ample, the preservations of solid contents are the advance requirements to achieve future application of industrial wastewaters in the advance recovery of phosphorus, preservation of microplastics, micropollutants elimination, and disinfection. While in the disposal or recycling process of sewage sludge or during wastewater treatment methods, the questions regarding the protection of water bodies, soil, human health, and resources should always be kept in mind.

Currently, wastewater treatment plants (WWTPs) have become system service providers—from just treating wastewaters, which includes treatment of wastewater/drainage for settlements, to being a service for water bodies by interaction with the energy industry. Now it has become a cross-linking system among wastewater treatment, waste and energy management, urban drainage, and agricultural land. In the future, the cooperation effects of these will benefit in a way that the WWTPs will become the primary component in the supply and disposal of arrangement systems.

# Bibliography

Ahmad A., Khan N., Giri B.S., Chowdhary P., Chaturvedi P. (2020) Removal of methylene blue dye using rice husk, cow dung and sludge biochar: characterization, application, and kinetic studies. *Bioresour. Technol.*, https://doi.org/10.1016/j.biortech.2020.123202.

Ahmed Al D., Govindrajan L., Talebi S., Al-Rajhi S., Al-Barwani T., AlBulashi Z. (2012) *Cultivation and Characterization of Microalgae for Wastewater Treatment.* World Congress on Engineering, Vol. 1, London, UK, ISBN: 978-988-19251-3-8.

Anjaneyulu Y., Sreedhara Chryz N., Samuel Suman Ra D. (2005) Decolorization of industrial effluents-available methods and emerging technologies- a review. *Rev. Environ. Sci. Bio/Technol.*, https://doi.org/10.100/s11157-005-1246-z.

Bai Y., Liang J., Liu R., Hu C., Qu J. (2014) Metagenomic analysis reveals microbial diversity and function in the rhizosphere soil of a constructed wetland. *Environ. Technol.* 35(20), 2521–2527.

Bai Y., Sun Q., Xing R., Wen D., Tang X. (2010) Removal of pyridine and quinoline by bio-zeolite composed of mixed degrading bacteria and modified zeolite. *J. Hazard. Mater.* 181, 916–922.

Bai Y., Sun Q., Zhao C., Wen D., Tang X. (2009) Simultaneous biodegradation of pyridine and quinoline by two mixed bacterial strains. *Appl. Microbiol. Biotechnol.* 82, 963–973.

Belinda S.M.S., Stacey L.L. (2011) An energy evaluation of coupling nutrient removal from wastewater with algal biomass production. *Appl. Energy* 88, 3499–3506.

Biermann C.J. (1993) *Essentials of Pulping and Papermaking.* Academic Press, Inc., San Diego, CA.

Blanco A., Negro C., Monte C., Fuente E., Tijero J. (2004) The challenges of sustainable papermaking. *Environ. Sci. Technol.* 38(21), 414A–420A. doi: 10.1021/es040654y.

Boman B., Ek M., Heyman W., Frostell B. (1991) Membrane filtration combined with biological treatment for purification of bleach plant effluents. *Water Sci. Technol.* 24(3/4), 219–228.

Bond R.G., Straub C.P., Prober H. (1974) *Wastewater Treatment and Disposal.* CRC Press.

Boon N., Goris J., De Vos P., Verstraete W., Top E.M. (2000) Bioaugmentation of activated sludge by an indigenous 3-chloroaniline-degrading *Comamonas testosteroni* strain, I2gfp. *Appl. Environ. Microbiol.* 66, 2906–2913.

Bouchez T., Patureau D., Dabert P., Juretschko S., Dore J., Delgenes P., Moletta R., Wagner M. (2000) Ecological study of a Bioaugmentation failure. *Environ. Microbiol.* 2, 179–190.

Boudh S., Chowdhary P., Hare V. Singh J.S., Seneviratne G. (eds). (2019) Agro-Environmental sustainability, volume 1: managing crop health. *Environ. Earth Sci.* 78, 655. https://doi.org/10.1007/s12665-019-8663-8.

Brault J.L., Degrement A. (1991) *Water Treatment Handbook.* Degremont, France.

BREF (2015) Best available techniques (BAT) reference document for the production of pulp, paper and board. JRC Science and Policy Reports, Industrial Emissions Directive 2010/75/EU, Integrated Pollution Prevention and Control.

Breithaupt H. (2006) The costs of REACH. *EMBO Rep.* 7, 968–971.

Burdon F.J., Munz N.A., Reyes M., Focks A., Joss A., Rasanen K. (2019) Agriculture versus wastewater pollution as drivers of macro invertebrate community structure in streams. *Sci. Total Environ.* 659, 1256–1265.

Burdon F.J., Reyes M., Alder A.C., Joss A., Ort C., Rasanen K. (2016) Environmental context and magnitude of disturbance influence trait-mediated community responses to wastewater in streams. *Ecol. Evol.* 6(12), 3923–3939.

Central Pollution Control Board. (2003) Chapter on corporate responsibility for environmental protection, distillery. Available from: http://www.cpcb.nic.in/Charter/charter5.htm.

Chambers P.A., Allard M., Walker S., Marsalek J., Lawrence J., Servos M. (1997) Impacts of municipal wastewater effluents on Canadian waters: a review. *Water Qual. Res. J.* 32(4), 659–714.

Chandra R., Chaudhary S. (2013) Persistent organic pollutants in environment and health hazards. *Int. J. Bioassays* 2(09), 1232–1238.

Chandra R., Chowdhary P. (2015). Properties of bacterial laccases and their application in bioremediation of industrial wastes. *Environ. Sci. Processes Impacts* 17, 326–342.

Chen M., Fan R., Zou W., Zhou H., Tan Z., Li X. (2016) Bioaugmentation for treatment of full-scale diethyleneglycol monobutyl ether (DGBE) wastewater by *Serratia* sp. BDG-2. *J. Hazard. Mater.* 309, 20–26.

Chopra A.K., Singh P.P. (2012) Removal of color, COD and lignin from pulp and paper mill effluent by *Phanerochaete chrysosporium* and *Aspergillus fumigates. J. Chem. Pharm. Res.* 4(10), 4522–4532.

Chowdhary P., Raj A., Bharagava R.N. (2018b) Environmental pollution and health hazards from distillery wastewater and treatment approaches to combat the environmental threats: a review. *Chemosphere* 194, 229–246.

Chowdhary P., Hare V., Raj A. (2018c) Book review: environmental pollutants and their bioremediation approaches. *Front. Bioeng. Biotechnol.* 6, 193. doi: 10.3389/fbioe.2018.00193.

Chowdhary P., Raj A., Bharagava R.N. (2017c) Environmental pollution and health hazards from distillery wastewater and treatment approaches to combat the environmental threats: a review. *Chemosphere* 194, 229–246.

Chowdhary P., Bharagava R.N. (2019) Toxicity, beneficial aspects and treatment of alcohol industry wastewater. In Bharagava R., Chowdhary P. (eds) *Emerging and Eco-Friendly Approaches for Waste Management.* Springer, Singapore.

Chowdhary P., Bharagava R.N. (2020a) Green technologies and environmental sustainability *Environ. Dev. Sustain.* 22, 2699–2701. https://doi.org/10.1007/s10668-018-00304.

Chowdhary P., Hare V., Mani S., Singh A.K., Zainith S., Raj A., Pandit S. (2020b) Recent advancement in the biotechnological application of lignin peroxidase and its future prospects. In Chowdhary P., Raj A., Verma D., Akhter Y. (eds) *Microorganisms for Sustainable Environment and Health*, 1–16.

Chowdhary P., More N., Raj A., Bharagava R.N. (2017) Characterization and identification of bacterial pathogens from treated tannery wastewater. *Microbiol. Res. Int.* 5(3), 30–36.

Chowdhary P., Sammi S.R., Pandey R., Kaithwas G., Raj A., Singh J., Bharagava R.N. (2020c) Bacterial degradation of distillery wastewater pollutants and their metabolites characterization and its toxicity evaluation by using *Caenorhabditis elegans* as terrestrial test models, Chemosphere. https://doi.org/10.1016/j.chemosphere.2020.127689.

Chowdhary P., Shukla G., Raj G., et al. (2019) Microbial manganese peroxidase: a ligninolytic enzyme and its ample opportunities in research. *SN Appl. Sci.* 1, 45. https://doi.org/10.1007/s42452-018-0046-3.

Chowdhary P., Yadav A., Singh R., Chandra R., Singh D.P., Raj A., Bharagava R.N. (2018a) Stress response of *Triticum aestivum* L. and *Brassica juncea* L. against heavy metals growing at distillery and tannery wastewater contaminated site. *Chemosphere* 206, 122–131.

Chowdhury M., Mostafa M.G., Biswas T.K. (2013) Treatment of leather industries effluents by filtration and coagulation process. *Water Res. Ind.* 3, 11–22.

Crites R., Tchobanoglous G. (1998) *Small and Decentralized Wastewater Management Systems*. McGraw-Hill, Boston, MA.

Crittenden J.C., Hu S., Hand D.W., Green S.A. (1999) A kinetic model for $H_2O_2$/UV process in a completely mixed batch reactor. *Water Res.* 33, 2315–2328.

Deniz I., Kirci H., Ates S. (2004) Optimisation of wheat straw *Triticum durum* kraft pulping. *Indust. Crops Prod.* 19(3), 237–243. doi: 10.1016/j.indcrop.2003.10.011.

Dey S., Islam A. (2015) A review on textile wastewater characterization in Bangladesh. *Resour. Environ.* 3(1), 15–44.

Dixit R., Wasiullah W., Malaviya D., Pandiyan K., Singh U.B., Sahu A., Paul D. (2015) Bioremediation of heavy metals from soil and aquatic environment: an overview of principles and criteria of fundamental processes. *Sustainability* 7(2), 2189–2212.

Doke K.M., Khan E.M., Rapolu J., Shaikh A. (2011) Physico-chemical analysis of sugar industry effluent and its effect on seed germination of *Vigna angularis, Vigna cylindrical* and *Sorghum cernum*. *Ann. Environ. Sci.*, 5, 7–11.

Dsikowitzky L., Schwarzbauer J. (2013) Organic contaminants from industrial wastewaters: identification, toxicity and fate in the environment. In Lichtfouse E., Schwarzbauer J., Robert D .(eds) *Pollutant Diseases, Remediation and Recycling*. Springer, Cham, pp 45–101. Environmental chemistry for a sustainable world.

Fan L., Liu D.Q., Zhu S.N., Mai J.X., Ni J.R. (2008) Degradation characteristics of bromoamine acid by*Sphingomonas* sp. FL. *Huan Jing KeXue* 29, 2618–2623.

Fan L., Ni J., Wu Y., Zhang Y. (2009) Treatment of bromoamine acid wastewater using combined process of micro-electrolysis and biological aerobic filter. *J. Hazard. Mater.* 162, 1204–1210.

Fan L., Zhu S., Liu D., Ni J. (2008) Decolorization mechanism of 1-amino-4-bromoanthraquinone-2-sulfonic acid using *Sphingomonas herbicidovorans* FL. *Dyes Pigments* 78, 34–38.

Fang F., Han H., Zhao Q., Xu C., Zhang L. (2013) Bioaugmentation of biological contact oxidation reactor (BCOR) with phenol-degrading bacteria for coal gasification wastewater (CGW) treatment. *Bioresour. Technol.* 150, 314–320.

Fontes A.G., Angelesvargas M., Fernandez J.M., et al. (1987) Factors affecting the production of biomass by a nitrogen-fixing blue-green alga in outdoor culture. *Biomass* 13(1), 33–43.

Garg S.K., Tripathi M. (2011) Strategies for decolorization and detoxification of pulp and paper mill effluent. In Whitacre D.M. (ed) *Reviews of Environmental Contamination and Toxicology*, 212, 113–136. doi: 10.1007/978-1-4419-8453-1_4.

Gartiser S., Hafner C., Hercher C., Kronenberger-Schafer K., Paschke A. (2010a) Whole effluent assessment of industrial wastewater for determination of BAT compliance. Part 1: paper manufacturing industry. *Environ. Sci. Pollut. Res.* 17, 856–865.

Hare V., Chowdhary P. (2019). Changes in growth responses in rice plants grown in the arsenic affected area: implication of As resistant microbes in mineral content and translocation. *SN Appl. Sci.* 1, 882. https://doi.org/10.1007/s42452-019-0945-y.

Hare V., Chowdhary P., Baghel V.S. (2017). Influence of bacterial strains on *Oryza sativa* grown under arsenic tainted soil: accumulation and detoxification response. *Plant Physiol. Biochem.* 119, 93–102.

Hare V., Chowdhary P., Kumar B., Sharma D.C., Baghel V.S. (2019) Arsenic toxicity and its remediation strategies for fighting the environmental threat. In Bharagava R., Chowdhary P. (eds) *Emerging and Eco-Friendly Approaches for Waste Management*. Springer, Singapore.

Hare V., Chowdhary P., Singh A.K. (2020) Arsenic toxicity: adverse effect and recent advance in microbes mediated bioremediation. In Chowdhary P., Raj A., Verma D., Akhter Y. (eds) *Microorganisms for Sustainable Environment and Health*, 53–80.

Herrero M., Stuckey D.C. (2015) Bioaugmentation and its application in wastewater treatment: a review. *Chemosphere* 140, 119–128.

Hossain K., Ismail N. (2015) Bioremediation and detoxification of pulp and paper mill effluent: a review. *Res. J. Environ. Toxicol.* 9(3), 113–134. doi:10.3923/rjet. 2015.113.134.

HSRC (2005) Hazardous Substances Research Centre/south and south west outreach program. Environmental hazards of the textile industry. Environmental update #24, Business week.

Igbinosa E.O., Okoh A.I. (2009) Impact of discharged wastewater effluents on the physico-chemical qualities of a receiving watershed in a typical rural community. *I. J. Environ. Sci. Technol.* 6(2), 175–182. doi: 10.1007/BF03327619.

Ince B.K., Zeynep C., Ince O. (2011) *Pollution Prevention in the Pulp and Paper Industries, Environmental Management in Practice*. Broniewicz E. (ed), InTech, China.

Kabeer R., Varghese R., Kannan V.M., Thomas J.R., Poulose S.V. (2014) Rhizosphere bacterial diversity and heavy metal accumulation in *Nymphaea pubescens* in aid of phytoremediation potential. *J. BioSci. Biotech.* 3(1), 89–95.

Kabra A.N., Khandare R.V., Govindwar S.P. (2012) Development of a bioreactor for remediation of textile effluent dye mixture: a plant-bacterial synergistic strategy. *Water Res.* 47, 1036–1048.

Kadirvelu K., Thamaraiselvi K., Namasivayam C. (2001) Removal of heavy metals from industrial wastewaters by adsorption onto activated carbon prepared from an agricultural solid waste. *Biores. Technol.* 76(1), 63–65.

Kalogerakis N. (2016) Bioaugmentation - is it really needed for the bioremediation of contaminated sites? Available online: http://www.srcosmos.gr/srcosmos/showpub. aspx?aa=8113 (accessed on 23 June 2016).

Kamali M., Khodaparast Z. (2015) Review on recent developments on pulp and paper mill wastewater treatment. *Ecotoxicol. Environ. Safety* 114, 326–342.

Karin L. (2006) Wastewater treatment with microalgae - a literature review. *VATTEN* 62, 31–38.

Kendrick M. (2011) *Algal Bioreactors for Nutrient Removal and Biomass Production during the Tertiary Treatment of Domestic Sewage.* Loughborough University Institutional Repository.

Kharche V.K., Desai V.N., Pharande A.L. (2011) Effect of sewage irrigation on soil properties, essential nutrients and pollutant element status of soils and plants in a vegetable growing area around Ahmednagar city in Maharashtra. *J. Indian Soc. Soil Sci.* 59(2), 177–184.

Kochany J. (2007) Wastewater treatment by membrane technology. *Onestoga-Rovers Assoc.* 7(3).

Latorre A., Malmqvist A., Lacorte S., Welander T., Barcelo D. (2007) Evaluation of the treatment efficiencies of paper mill whitewaters in terms of organic composition and toxicity. *Environ. Pollut.* 147(3), 648–655. doi:10.1016/j.envpol.2006.09.015.

Lee G., Zhang Y., Shao S. (2014) International conference on environment systems science and engineering (ESSE 2014) study on recycling alkali from the wastewater of textile mercerization process by nanofiltration. *IERI Procedia* 9, 71–76.

Lehto J., Alen R. (2015) Organic materials in black liquors of soda-AQ pulping of hot-water-extracted birch *(Betulapendula)* sawdust. *Holzforschung* 69(3), 257–264. doi: 10.1515/hf-2014-0094.

Liang T., Wang L. (2015) An environmentally safe and nondestructive process for bleaching birch veneer with peracetic acid. *J. Clean. Prod.* 92, 37–43.

Liu X., Chen Y., Zhang X., Jiang X., Wu S., Shen J., Sun X., Li J., Lu L., Wang L. (2015) Aerobic granulation strategy for Bioaugmentation of a sequencing batch reactor (SBR) treating high strength pyridine wastewater. *J. Hazard. Mater.* 295, 153–160.

Loffler F.E., Ritalahti K.M., Zinder S.H. (2013) Dehalococcoides and reductive de-chlorination of chlorinated solvents. In Ward C.H. (ed) *Bioaugmentation for Groundwater Remediation.* Springer Science and Business Media, New York, NY, 39–88.

Lofrano G., Brown J. (2010) Wastewater management through the ages: a history of mankind. *Sci. Total Environ.* 408, 5254–5264.

Lofrano G., Meric S., Balci G.E.Z., Orhon D. (2013) Chemical and biological treatment technologies for leather tannery chemicals and wastewaters: a review. *Sci. Total Environ.* 461–462, 265–281.

Luan H., Diao F., Peabody N.C., White B.H. (2012) Command and compensation in a neuromodulatory decision network. *J. Neurosci.* 32(3), 880–889.

Magdum S.S., Minde G.P., Kalyanraman V. (2013) Rapid determination of indirect cod and polyvinyl alcohol from textile desizing wastewater. *Pollut. Res.* 32, 515–519.

Mallevialle J., Odendall P.E., Wiesner M.R. (1996) *Water Treatment Membrane Processes.* McGraw-Hill, New York.

Mani S., Bharagava R.N. (2016) Exposure to crystal violet, its toxic, genotoxic and carcinogenic effects on environment and its degradation and detoxification for environmental safety. *Rev. Environ. Contam. Toxicol.* 273, 71–104.

Mani S., Chowdhary P., Bharagava R.N. (2019) Textile wastewater dyes: toxicity profile and treatment approaches. In Bharagava R., Chowdhary P. (eds) *Emerging and Eco-Friendly Approaches for Waste Management.* Springer, Singapore.

Manisankar P., Rani C., Viswanathan S. (2004) Effect of halides in the electrochemical treatment of distillery effluent. *Chemosphere.* 57(8), 961–966.

Mattes T.E., Alexander A.K., Coleman N.V. (2010) Aerobic biodegradation of the chloroethenes: pathways, enzymes, ecology, and evolution. *FEMS Microbiol. Rev.* 34, 445–475.

Matthew N.C. (2008) Biodiesel: algae as a renewa ble source for liquid fuel. *Guelph Eng. J.* 1, 2–7. ISSN: 19161107.

McCubbin N., Folke J.N. (1993) A review of literature on pulp and paper mill effluent characteristics in the peace and Athabasca river basins. In Northern River Basins Study Project Report No. 15, N. McCubbin Consultants Inc., Edmonton.

Megharaj M., Ramakrishnan B., Venkateswarlu K., Sethunanthan N., Naidu R. (2011) Bioremediation approaches for organic pollutants: a critical perspective. *Environ. Int.* 37(8), 1362–1375.

Melamane X.L., Strong P.J., Burgess J.E. (2007) Treatment of wine distillery wastewater: a review with emphasis on anaerobic membrane reactors. *S. Afr. J. Enol. Vitic.* 28(1), 25–36.

Miao Q., Huang L.L., Chen L.H. (2013) Advances in the control of dissolved and colloidal substances present in papermaking processes: a brief review. *Bio Resourc.* 8(1), 1431–1455. doi: 10.15376/biores.8.1.1431-1455.

Mishra S., Chowdhary P., Bharagava R.N. (2019) Conventional methods for the removal of industrial pollutants, their merits and demerits. In Bharagava R., Chowdhary P. (eds) *Emerging and Eco-Friendly Approaches for Waste Management.* Springer, Singapore.

Mohana S., Bhavik K.A., Madamwar D. (2009) Distillery spent wash: treatment technologies and potential applications. *J. Hazard Mater.* 163(1), 12–25.

Momba M., Tyafa Z., Makala N., Brouckaert B., Obi C. (2006) Safe drinking water still a dream in rural areas of South Africa. *Case Study Eastern Cape Province.Water SA* 32, 47864.

Mounteer A.H., Souza L.C., Silva C.M. (2007a) Potential for enhancement of aerobic biological removal of recalcitrant organic matter in bleached pulp mill effluents. *Environ. Technol.* 28(2), 157–164. doi: 10.1080/09593332808618775.

Muhamad M.H., Abdullah S.R.S., Mohamad A.B., Rahman R.A., Kadhum A.A.H. (2012a) Kinetic evaluation and process performance of a pilot GAC-SBBR system treating recycled paper industry wastewater. *Environ. Eng. Manag. J.* 11(4), 829–839.

Nadal M., Schuhmacher M., Domingo J.L. (2004) Metal Pollution of soils and vegetation in an area with petrochemical industry. *Sci. Total Environ.* 321(1–3), 59–69.

Omatoyo K.D., Trina H., Innocent U., Benjamin G., John W., Qiong Z., Sarina E. (2013) Wastewater use in algae production for generation of renewable resources: a review and preliminary result. *Aquat. Biosyst.* 9, 2.

Pandey A., Singh P., Iyengar L. (2007) Bacterial decolorization and degradation of azo dyes. *Int. Biodeterior. Biodegrad.* 59, 73–84.

Pant D., Adholeya A. (2007b) Enhanced production of ligninolytic enzymes and decolorization of molassed distillery wastewater by fungi under solid state fermentation. *Biodegradation.* 18, 647–659.

Park D., Lee D.S., Kim Y.M., Park J.M. (2008) Bioaugmentation of cyanide-degrading microorganisms in a full-scale cokes wastewater treatment facility. *Bioresour. Technol.* 99, 2092–2096.

Pokhrel D., Viraraghavan T. (2004) Treatment of pulp and paper mill wastewater - a review. *Sci. Total Environ.* 333, 37–58. doi: 10.1016/j.scitotenv.2004.05.017.

Power E.A., Boumphrey R.S. (2004) International trends in bioassay use for effluent management: UK DTA demonstration programme. *Ecotoxicology* 13(5), 377–398.

Providenti M.A., Lee H., Trevors J.T. (1993) Selected factors limiting the microbial degradation of recalcitrant compounds. *J. Ind. Microbiol.* 12, 379–395.

Puyol D., Monsalvo V.M., Sanchis S., Sanz J.L., Mohedano A.F., Rodriguez J.J. (2015) Comparison of bioaugmented EGSB and GAC-FBB reactors and their combination with aerobic SBR for the abatement of chlorophenols. *Chem. Eng. J.* 259, 277–285.

Quan X., Shi H., Liu H., Lv P.,Qian Y. (2004) Enhancement of 2,4-dichlorophenol degradation in conventional activated sludge systems bioaugmented with mixed special culture. *Water Res.* 38, 245–253.

Ravikumar R., Saravanan R., Vasanthi N.S., Swetha J., Akshaya N., Rajthilak M., Kannan K.P. (2007) Biodegradation and decolorization of biomethanated distillery spent wash. *Indian J. Sci. Technol.* 1(2), 1–6.

Rein M.J. (2005) Co-pigmentation reactions and color stability of berry anthocyanins (dissertation). EKT series 1331. *University of Helsinki, Department of Applied Chemistry and Microbiology.* 88+34 pp.

Satyawali Y., Balakrishanan M. (2007) Wastewater treatment in molasses-based alcohol distilleries for COD and color removal: a review. *J. Environ. Manage.* 86, 481–497.

Savant D.V., Abdul-Rahman R., Ranade D.R. (2006) Anaerobic degradation of adsorbable organic halides (AOX) from pulp andpaper industry wastewater. *Bioresour. Technol.* 97(9), 1092–1104. doi: 10.1016/j.biortech.2004.12.013.

Schaum C., Cornel P. (2016) Wastewater treatment of the future: health, water and resource protection. *Aust. Water Waste Manage.* 3–4. doi:10.1007/s00506-016-0296-5.

Schaum C., Fundneider T., Cornel P. (2015a) Analysis of methane emissions from-digested sludge. *Water Sci. Technol.* doi: 10.2166/wst.2015.644.

Sekaran G., Karthikeyan S., Nagalakshmi C., Mandal A.B. (2013) Integrated *Bacillus* sp. immobilized cell reactor and *Synechocystis* sp. algal reactor for the treatment of tannery wastewater. *Environ. Sci. Pollut. Res.* 20, 281–291.

Semrany S., Favier L., Djelal H., Taha S., Amrane A. (2012) Bioaugmentation: possible solution in the treatment of Bio-Refractory Organic Compounds (Bio-ROCs). *Biochem. Eng. J.* 69, 75–86.

Sen B., Alp M.T., Sonmez F., Kocer M.A.T., Canpolat O. (2013) Relationship of algae to water pollution and waste water treatment. *Wastewater Treat.*, 335–354.

Shah D.G. (2007) Pharma policy-crippling draft proposals. *The Hindu Survey of Indian Industry*, 254–255.

Singh C., Chowdhary P., Singh J.S., Chandra R. (2016). Pulp and paper mill wastewater and coliform as health hazards: a review. *Microbiol. Res. Int.* 4(3), 28–39.

Singh P., Srivastava A. (2014) Enzymatic colour removal of pulp and paper mill effluent by different fungal strains. *Int. J. Pharm. Bio. Sci.* 5(3), 773–783.

Sitarek K., Gromadzinska J., Lutz P., Stetkiewicz J., Swiercz R., Wasowicz W. (2012) Fertility and developmental toxicity studies of diethylene glycol monobutyl ether (DGBE) in rats. *Int. J. Occup. Med. Environ. Health* 25, 404–417.

Stroo H.F., Leeson A., Ward C.H. (2013) *Bioaugmentation for Groundwater Remediation.* Springer Science and Business Media, New York, NY, 389.

Tielbaard M., Wilson T., Feldbaumer E., Driessen W. (2002) Full-scale anaerobic treatment experiences with pulp mill evaporator condensates. Proc. TAPPI Environmental Conf., TAPPI Press, Atlanta.

Travieso L., Benitez F., Dupeyron R. (1999) Algae growth potential measurement in distillery wastes. *Bull. Environ. Contam. Toxicol.* 62, 483–489.

Tuo B.H., Yan J.B., Fan B.A., Yang Z.H., Liu J.Z. (2012) Biodegradation characteristics and Bioaugmentation potential of a novel quinoline-degrading strain of *Bacillus* sp. isolated from petroleum-contaminated soil. *Bioresour. Technol.* 107, 55–60.

Ugurlu M., Karaoglu M.H. (2009) Removal of AOX, total nitrogen and chlorinated lignin from bleached kraft mill effluents by UV oxidation in the presence of hydrogen peroxide utilizing TiO as photocatalyst. *Environ. Sci. Pollution Res.* 16(3), 265–273. doi:10.1007/s11356-008-0044-x.

Vepsalainen M., Selin J., Rantala P., Pulliainen M., Sarkka H., Kuhmonen K., Bhatnagar A., Sillanpaa M. (2011) Precipitation of dissolved sulphide in pulp and paper mill wastewater by electrocoagulation. *Environ. Technol.* 32(12), 1393–1400.

Wang J.H., He H.Z., Wang M.Z., Wang S., Zhang J., Wei W., Xu H.X., Lv Z.M., Shen D.S. (2013) Bioaugmentation of activated sludge with *Acinetobacter* sp. TW enhances nicotine degradation in a synthetic tobacco wastewater treatment system. *Bioresour. Technol.* 42C, 445–453.

Wang J., Liu G.F., Lu H., Jin R.F., Zhou J.T., Lei T.M. (2012) Biodegradation of Acid Orange 7 and its auto-oxidative decolorization product in membrane-aerated biofilm reactor. *Int. Biodeterior. Biodegrad.* 67, 73–77.

Wang M., Xu J., Wang J., Wang S., Feng H., Shentu J., Shen D. (2013) Differences between 4-fluoroanilinedegradation and autoinducer release by *Acinetobacter* sp. TW: implications for operating conditions in bacterial Bioaugmentation. *Environ. Sci. Pollut. Res. Int.* 20, 6201–6209.

Wang M., Yang G., Min H., Lv Z., Jia X. (2009) Bioaugmentation with the nicotine-degrading bacterium *Pseudomonas* sp. HF-1 in a sequencing batch reactor treating tobacco wastewater: degradation study and analysis of its mechanisms. *Water Res.* 43, 4187–4196.

Wang M.Z., Yang G.Q., Wang X., Yao Y.L., Min H., Lv Z.M. (2011) Nicotine degradation by two novel bacterial isolates of *Acinetobacter* sp. TW and *Sphingomonas* sp. TY and their responses in the presence of neonicotinoid insecticides. *World J. Microbiol. Biotechnol.* 27, 1633–1640.

Wen D., Zhang J., Xiong R., Liu R., Chen L. (2013) Bioaugmentation with a pyridine-degrading bacterium in a membrane bioreactor treating pharmaceutical wastewater. *J. Environ. Sci.* 25, 2265–2271.

WHO (2009) *Global Prevalence of Vitamin A Deficiency in Populations at Risk 1995–2005.* WHO Global Database on Vitamin A Deficiency, Geneva.

Wiesner M.R., Hackney J., Sethi S., Jacangelo J.G., Laine J.M. (1994) Cost estimates for membrane filtration and conventional treatment. *J. Am. Water Works Assoc.* 85(12), 33–41.

Willfor S., Sjoholm R., Laine C., Roslund M., Hemming J., Holmbom B. (2003) Characterisation of water-soluble galactoglucomannans from Norway spruce wood and thermomechanical pulp. *Carbohyd. Polym.* 52(2), 175–187. doi: 10.1016/S0144-8617(02)00288-6.

Wu J., Xiao Y.Z., Yu H.Q. (2005) Degradation of lignin in pulp mill wastewaters by white-rot fungi on biofilm. *Bioresour. Technol.* 96, 1357–1363.

Xin L., Guoyi L. (2015) *A Review: Pharmaceutical Wastewater Treatment Technology and Research in China.* Asia-Pacific Energy Equipment Engineering Research Conference, Zhuhai, 345–347.

Xu P., Ma W., Han H., Jia S., Hou B. (2015) Isolation of a naphthalene-degrading strain from activated sludge and Bioaugmentation with it in a MBR treating coal gasification wastewater. *Bull. Environ. Contam. Toxicol.* 94, 358–364.

Yafei S. (2014) Carbon dioxide bio-fixation and wastewater treatment via algae photochemical synthesis for biofuels production. *RSC Adv.* 4, 49672–49722.

Yang S.Y., Lou L.P., Wang K., Chen Y.X. (2006) Shift of initial mechanism in $TiO_2$-assisted photocatalytic process. *Appl. Catal. A.* 301, 152–157.

Yu Y. (2013) *Experimental on Pharmaceutical Tail Water before Biochemical Pretreatment.* Jilin University, Changchun, 12–19.

Zaharia C. (2009) A preliminary optimization study applied for a homogenous oxidation with hydrogen peroxide of an industrial wastewater. Proceeding of the 13th International Conference – Modern Technologies, Quality and Innovation – ModTech, New face of T.M.C.R., Iasi, Romania, 711–714.

Zainith S., Chowdhary P., Bharagava R.N. (2019) Recent advances in physico-chemical and biological techniques for the management of pulp and paper mill waste. In Bharagava R., Chowdhary P. (eds) *Emerging and Eco-Friendly Approaches for Waste Management.* Springer, Singapore.

Zhang Y., Chai L.Y., Yang Z.H., Tang C.J., Chen Y.H., Shi Y. (2013) Enhanced remediation of black liquor by activated sludge bioaugmented with a novel exogenous microorganism culture. *Appl. Microbiol. Biotechnol.* 97, 6525–6535.

Zhong W., Zhu C., Shu M., Sun K., Zhao L., Wang C., Ye Z., Chen J. (2010) Degradation of nicotine in tobacco waste extract by newly isolated *Pseudomonas* sp. ZUTSKD. *Bioresour. Technol.* 101, 6935–6941.

Zhou H., Smith D.W. (2002) Advanced technologies in water and wastewater treatment. *J. Environ. Eng. Sci.* 1, 247–264.

Zhu X., Liu R., Liu C., Chen L. (2015) Bioaugmentation with isolated strains for the removal of toxic and refractory organics from coking wastewater in a membrane bioreactor. *Biodegradation* 26, 465–474.

Zollinger H. (1987) *Colour Chemistry – Synthesis, Properties of Organic Dyes and Pigments.* VCH Publishers, New York, pp 92–100.

# Index

Note: Page numbers in **bold** represent tables.